FREE TO BE SLIM

Free to Be Slim

MARIE CHAPIAN & NEVA COYLE

KINGSWAY PUBLICATIONS

EASTBOURNE

Copyright © Marie Chapian & Neva Coyle 1979

First published in the USA by Bethany House Publishers,
Minneapolis, Minnesota

First British Edition 1985
Reprinted 1985
Reprinted 1986
Reprinted 1987
Reprinted 1989

ISBN 0 86065 344 7

Biblical quotations are from the New American
Standard Bible © The Lockman Foundation 1960, 1962, 1963,
1968, 1971, 1972, 1973

AV = Authorized Version (crown copyright)

Printed in Great Britain for
KINGSWAY PUBLICATIONS LTD
1 St. Anne's Rd, Eastbourne, E. Sussex BN21 3UN
Courier International Ltd, Tiptree, Essex
Typeset by Nuprint Services Ltd, Harpenden, Herts.

This book is dedicated
to your body

Contents

Introduction

Yesterday

At 28 years old, Neva Coyle weighed 17st 10lb. When people look at a 'before picture' of her, they can't believe it's the same person. Being almost 8st lighter, Neva is now an attractive, vibrant woman and the president and founder of Overeaters Victorious, in the United States.

One of the happiest experiences in her life was buying a size 12 skirt and throwing out her size 24 wardrobe.

'I just wanted to be *average*,' she says. 'I used to think I'd give anything just to be average.'

She remembers her many attempts to lose weight. 'I tried every diet known to mankind,' she says. 'All the weight-loss groups and clinics too. I'd lose weight and then regain it, plus more.'

Her motives for losing weight were varied. Maybe you will recognize some of them. She tried losing weight for her husband. She thought he deserved a slim wife, one he could be proud of. But after a while, she couldn't stick to the diet any longer. That ice-cream parlour up the road was just too irresistible, and the smell of pizza was more than she could take.

Unhappily, food had a stronger hold on her than her desire to please her husband.

She also tried to lose weight for her friends' sakes. She was singing in a church trio and the girls decided to buy matching dresses. Neva was disgraced and humiliated as they tried to squeeze her into a size 18 dress that she could barely get over her head. 'I'll lose weight for them,' she told herself. 'Then I'll fit into one of these shop-bought dresses!' (At her size, she had to make her own clothes.)

Not a strong enough motive. It didn't work. She gained weight instead.

She dieted for special occasions: weddings, special parties, and church meals. But she never quite made it. Eating was more important than the special event, just as eating was more important than her friends and loved ones.

Looking nice is a strong motive for many people. For the overeater it is not a motive, it is a wish. Wishing something and being motivated to bring it about are two different things.

Neva, like many other overeaters, tried dieting for herself. 'Do it because you like yourself,' the counsellors told her. The trouble was, she didn't like herself. Most obese people don't. You don't usually go out of your way for someone you don't like. And you're certainly not likely to give up something that you are passionately addicted to for someone you don't like. No, she couldn't lose weight, not even for her own self-esteem.

Desperately she sought to lose the weight, but didn't know how to do it without giving up what she loved the most: eating.

That was until she heard about by-pass surgery. She went into hospital on January 9th, 1972, and had a by-pass operation.

After this dangerous, painful and expensive surgery, she was horrified to discover that her dream of eating everything she wanted without getting fat did not come true after all. Although she lost weight initially, she soon began regaining. When she had gained 1½st she panicked. She had to do something. There *had* to be help somewhere, she told herself.

Then she did something radical. Something outrageous. She turned to God.

Two years after the by-pass surgery she was still suffering the after-effects of it. Worst of all, she wasn't even thin; in fact, she was still grossly overweight. She was broken-hearted, miserable and desperate.

Are you at the point of desperation yet? Are you fed up with yourself and the way you're treating your body? You don't have to be a victim of overeating any longer. You can be free!

For the eyes of the Lord move to and fro throughout the earth that He may strongly support those whose heart is completely His (2 Chron 16:9).

I will instruct you and teach you in the way which you should go; I will counsel you with My eye upon you (Ps 32:8).

The Lord longs to help you if you will permit him. He loves you dearly. You are very important to him and it is important to him that you be healthy in every area of your life. He waits to help you lose weight.

Since the day back in 1973 when Neva Coyle became committed to losing weight permanently, she has lost 8st and gained the attention of many. 'How did you do it?' people ask. 'Will it work for me?'

She has appeared on American television, and her story has been in newspapers across the United States, Canada and Europe.

In four years she went from being an unhappy, obese

housewife to an attractive director of an international organization showing others the way to being slim and God-centred eating.

To thousands of overweight men and women, Over-eaters Victorious offers hope and an answer to prayer in a dark and hopeless way of life, due to overeating.

When Neva Coyle cried out to God for help in her battle against overeating, she didn't imagine he would answer her prayers in such a dramatic way, as to make her instrumental in the answered prayers of thousands of others as well.

This book is not to promote Overeaters Victorious, but to share with you what Neva Coyle has learned and now teaches in order that you can lose weight and *keep it off*.

This is a book about success. The people whose examples appear here were once victims of emotional disturbances and neurotic behaviour. They were gorgers, bingers, gluttons; they craved and consumed junk foods and sugar until it not only poisoned their appearance, but their personalities and health as well. They were unhappy, sick and trapped.

If you are really serious about being right with God and if you mean business about pleasing him, living for him and eating for him, then he is ready to help you.

One last thing before you begin—at the end of most chapters in this book there is a prayer for you to pray. This is very important to do. Pray these prayers aloud (the more times the better). You will find a new strength and power in your life that you didn't know you could have through this victorious praying.

If you are tired of endless weight-loss schemes, diets and diet clubs, and if you truly want your body, as well as your soul and spirit, in line with God's will, then this book is the book for you.

God bless you!

One

Free To Be Slim

Carol was 6st 6lb overweight. She was lonely, angry and at the end of her tether. In her opinion, there was no answer to her weight problem. She agonized at being overweight but continued eating and going on food binges. She and two overweight friends often went out together and did something they called 'pigging out'. They went from restaurant to restaurant eating until they could barely walk. The next day Carol would suffer food hangover worse than a hangover due to alcohol.

Carol went on dozens of diets. She would lose a stone and gain two. Desperate and miserable, Carol cried out to God for help. Her small 5ft 1in frame weighed 15st.

Carol's life parallels the lives of thousands of other people who have never reached the fulfilment of their dream to be slim. Slim! Carol tried everything she could think of to become slim—diet pills, diet shots, diet chewing-gum, hypnosis, Weightwatchers, and diets! She had tried them all: the F-Plan diet, the grapefruit diet, the banana diet, the ice cream diet, the carbohydrate diet, the protein diet, the potato diet, the celery and carrot diet. She had taken liquid protein and lost 1st 6lb. (She put 2st 2lb back on and needed a week in hospital.) She tried Slender and other powdered protein drinks and only lost 5lb because she'd drink the protein drink and then eat a full meal. She fasted, lived on juices alone for weeks at a time, and even as a last resort tried acupuncture. When that didn't work, she opted for by-pass surgery. The surgeon told her she wasn't heavy enough. She needed to be 7st overweight and she was just under that.

A person is desperate when he pursues a painful and dangerous operation such as by-pass surgery which slices across the stomach, making a 15–18in incision to disconnect approximately 9ft of the small intestine, leaving the patient with 18in of functioning intestine. Side effects and complications are frequent. But still the drastic choice of by-pass surgery is appealing—a glutton's dream. 'I can eat as much as I want without gaining weight!'

Carol, however, didn't go through with the surgery. She heard a success story that changed her life. A woman had lost over 8st and she was helping countless others to lose weight too.

Carol decided to see what it was all about. She met the woman who had lost so much weight. 'I lost every pound with Jesus,' she confessed.

Carol was very interested. 'With—?'

'That's right. With Jesus,' Neva Coyle told her. 'Nothing else worked. Nothing. And I was pretty desperate. I mean, you're really desperate when you're willing to give up your life to be slim. And that's where I was when I had the by-pass surgery. Then after the surgery I started gaining again. I gained a stone and the scales were going up every day! It was then that I realized overeating was a spiritual problem. And if it's a spiritual problem, the answer has to be God.'

As she talked, Carol was impressed with this woman wearing a *belted* jacket and a skirt with *horizontal* stripes.

The following week Carol joined Overeaters Victorious, the weight-loss organization which had grown out of Neva Coyle's successful weight-loss methods.

Carol's story hasn't ended yet. She began attending the meetings, doing her homework, and the Lord began to answer her prayers. Each week at weigh-in time Carol recorded a new weight loss. In a matter of 6½ months, she had lost 5st. Her dream of being thin was almost realized. 'Like Neva, I just wanted to be *average*. I hated being called obese.'

Then Carol shares the most interesting part of all. 'Being slim is really almost a by-product of the real victory that has happened in my life,' she says. 'The real victory is the one over self and self-indulgence.'

Overeaters Victorious members share openly how God helped them overcome anger, fear, jealousy, loneliness and frustration through losing weight. Being slim for the first time in their lives is a dream come true, but even better is the fact that they are completely new people.

All things are possible in Christ, and that includes losing weight.

The aim of this book is to tell you how to lose weight *for ever*. If you follow the guidelines, you will become slim and stay slim. You will also learn a new way of life.

Overeating isn't something that affects only the body. It is intricately involved and intertwined with the emotions. It is the personality that produces the fat, in fact. Psychologists tell us that being overweight is often an indication of a maladjusted personality. Overeating, especially sweets, is often a response to feelings of inadequacy, depression, anger, fear, loneliness, fear of failure, anxiety and other debilitating emotions.

Overweight people use eating as an emotional outlet. Dr Charles S. Freed, an authority on obesity, explains, 'Anything that increases the overeater's emotional tension (such as sorrow, anxiety, nervousness or irritability) increases their desire for food,'[1]

Every successful Overeaters Victorious person will tell you how much *more* God did in his life than just remove extra weight.

If you're really serious about being right with God and if you mean business about pleasing him and living for him, now is the time to start.

For far too long Christians have been making excuses for destroying their bodies.

Being 1, 3 or 8st overweight is far more harmful than you may realize.

Dr Frederick J. Stare[2] of Harvard University's Nutrition Department says that even being a stone over normal weight can mean that you run the risk of dying 5 or 10 years sooner than you otherwise might. He says being a stone overweight is being in the 'alarm zone'.

Gorging on food wounds more than our bodies. Our souls are hurt too. Unfortunately, being obese seems to be acceptable. If there's a drug addict or an alcoholic in the church, everybody can plainly see someone with a serious problem. But the obese person, addicted to gluttony, is regarded as normal.

Is obesity normal in the eyes of the Lord? Compulsive acts without evidence of disease fall under the category of psycho-neurosis. Overeating is a compulsive act. Jesus went to the cross so that his people no longer need be the victims of compulsive acts. We need to ask ourselves, then, 'Is overeating sin?'

'Ouch!' you say. 'I've never considered my overweight *sin*! I mean, I'm free to be who I am in the Lord. He loves me just the way I am! Fat or thin, I'm his and he loves me.'

---

[1] Kordel, Lelord, *Eat and Grow Slender*. (Manor Books, Inc.) 1962
[2] Ibid.

What shall we say then? Are we to continue in sin that grace might increase? May it never be! (Rom 6:1–2).

The overweight person may say the truth with his mouth, but he doesn't really believe he is totally loved. That's one of the reasons for overeating. Food takes the role of the comforter.

The overweight person may also say, 'I love the Lord and I want to serve and obey him!'

And that's the key to dynamic living and power-obedience. The Bible tells us in Galatians 5:23 that evidence of the Holy Spirit's working in our lives is self-control. Obeying the Lord means hearing him when he says, 'Don't eat that!' and then obeying.

Would we rather overeat than allow the Holy Spirit to hold the reins of our appetites?

Lust for food will never be satisfied. Unbridled lust is sinful, and lust for food is as sinful as unbridled physical lust for someone's body. Eating to gain a false sense of security is a false motive because only God gives us true security and safety.

Our first step, then, towards becoming slim and staying slim is to consider the commitments before us. It's a wonderful and powerful commitment, one that will have a dynamic effect on us for the rest of our lives.

Are you ready?

Two

Making a Commitment

The Holy Spirit longs to be the guiding force in your life, and longs to fill every need you have.

Ask yourself this question: 'Will I allow the Holy Spirit to take over my eating habits?'

If you have answered 'Yes', you're ready to begin.

You are now about to learn how to bring your body into control by training your flesh in the power of the Holy Spirit.

Don't be afraid. With God you won't fail. In the past you may have failed at losing weight; in fact, you may have even failed when you tried losing weight with the Lord. Remember, God is a patient and forgiving God. He is right beside you at this moment—ready to begin work with you on your eating habits.

How much do you eat?

If you are eating more than your body requires, you are putting more into it than God intended it to hold. If you are hungry for more than your body needs, it's not food you're hungering for.

We are made of body, soul and spirit. In order to be rightly aligned with the will of God, your *spirit* should

18

be the controlling force in your life. Your human spirit, indwelled and empowered by the Holy Spirit of God, then is able to be in constant communion with God. You are able to hear his voice, understand his word, obey him in all things. Your body and soul respond to the power of God in your spirit.

If your *body* tells your soul and spirit what to do, you're out of order and you will fail.

If your *soul* is in control, and this is the area most people are led by, you are also out of the will of God. Your soul is comprised of intellect, emotion and will. If your emotions lead your life, you are in a sorry state, vulnerable to any circumstance or event. If your intellect alone guides your life, you are without the wisdom of God who is all wise. If your will directs you, you are at best stubborn.

When you are filled with food and still hungry, you are receiving some very direct signals that your inner being is longing for more than food. Filling your stomach will not satisfy that longing and the more you eat, the fatter and hungrier you'll be. The person who says, 'I don't eat out of deep needs. I eat because I enjoy food,' is really saying, 'I don't want God to tamper with my appetite.' That person may just be refusing to discipline his/her eating habits or exercise the godly fruit of self-control.

God's promise for success

Just before God gave Moses the law, he showed him the importance of a covenant. It was important in order to be successful, or to prosper. 'Prosper' means to be successful, to thrive. (It is the overweight person's goal to prosper in his/her efforts to lose weight!)

God promised prosperity or success for keeping a covenant.

So keep the words of this covenant to do them, that you may prosper in all that you do (Deut 29:9).

You enter into a covenant with God to lose weight his way. You know all too well that your own efforts to lose weight will bring failure and disappointment. But God will not disappoint you. Be assured that God is joining *with* you. A covenant is something requiring more than one. God will not only encourage you on your way to being slim, he will also show you the way!

You stand today...before the Lord your God...that you may enter into the covenant with the Lord your God, and into His oath which the Lord your God is making with you today, in order that He may establish you today as His people and that He may be your God, just as He spoke to you and as He swore to your fathers, to Abraham, Isaac, and Jacob (Deut 29:10, 12, 13).

The commitment

Before you begin to lose weight, carefully and prayerfully make a decision to commit yourself wholly to doing it God's way. When you come to him on his terms, seeking his ways, asking his guidance, he will guide, comfort, encourage, strengthen and see to it that you're successful.

For this commandment which I command you today is not too difficult for you, nor is it out of reach (Deut 30:11).

You agree *with* him to go on a definite retraining course. You agree *with* him to see it through, to remain faithful. Notice we use the word 'faithful' but we do not use the word 'diet'. Overeaters Victorious do not learn how to diet. We learn how to *eat*. Every overweight person already knows how to diet and probably knows a hundred different diets. We are not dieting; we are training our eating habits through the power of the Holy Spirit and the word of God.

> But the word is very near you, in your mouth and in your heart, that you may observe it (Deut 30:14).

You can be faithful fo him and to his word if you will connect your will to his. He has a great purpose for your life and his purpose always requires obedience on your part. In order to be obedient you have to be faithful.

> See, I have set before you today life and prosperity, and death and adversity; in that I command you today to love the Lord your God, to walk in His ways and to keep His commandments and His statutes and His judgments, that you may live and multiply, and that the Lord your God may bless you in the land where you are entering to possess it (Deut 30:15–16).

God promises you that you will be blessed if you will listen to him, walk his ways and keep his commandments. (Those commandments may come in the form of a loud inner voice, for example, 'Don't eat that!' while you're reaching for the biscuit tin.)

You lose the promise by turning away, by choosing not to obey him.

> But if your heart turns away and you will not obey, but are drawn away and worship other gods and serve them, I declare to you today that you shall surely perish. You shall not prolong *your* days in the land where you are crossing the Jordan to enter and possess it (Deut 30:17–18).

Think of your 'promised land' as a slim body. You can enter into your promised land and enjoy the fullness of life that God gives to those who are obedient, or you can forfeit it.

... I have set before you life and death, the blessing and the curse. So choose life in order that you may live, you and your descendants (Deut 30:19).

How do we choose life? He gives some specific directions in the next verse:

By loving the Lord your God, by obeying His voice, and by holding fast to Him; for this is your life and the length of your days (Deut 30:20).

The Lord urges you to choose life. The choice, now, is yours.

If you don't have an intimate, personal relationship with Jesus Christ, you can. Give your life to him, making him the Lord of your life. He came to this world as the Son of God, to die on the cross, so that you and I could be forgiven of all sins and live a life of victory over negative and destructive forces. When he is your Lord and Saviour, you have the Holy Spirit of God dwelling within your spirit to link your life with the power of heaven and eternity. It is the Holy Spirit who guides, instructs, comforts and helps you as you lose weight.

What does commitment really mean?

What does the word 'commitment' mean to you? Two definitions of the word are 'a pledge' or 'the state of being bound emotionally or intellectually to some course of action'. In order to live a dynamic Christian life in God, you need commitment. It's not something to take lightly.

If you are willing to give Jesus lordship over every area of your life, including what you eat, you must commit yourself to this idea.

Make a covenant with the Lord today regarding total commitment to him and his will. Then make a commitment regarding losing weight. A covenant is a *binding agreement*, and your commitment to the Lord requires this covenant.

You are agreeing and binding yourself to the Lord, not to anyone or anything else. Your commitment is to Jesus.

Your commitment to losing weight and getting your body into good shape is important. If it is sincere, you will succeed. God promises you that.

PRAYER

Father, in the name of Jesus, I make Jesus the Lord of my life. I give my body, soul and spirit to you now. I receive Jesus as my Saviour and I choose to live my life now by the power of the Holy Spirit.

I make a commitment to you, Lord, regarding my eating habits. I choose to put you in the position of Lord over every area of my life, particularly in the area of eating.

I choose to love you, to obey your voice and to hold fast to you because you have said this is my life and the length of my days. I choose the blessing of obedience.

In Jesus' name, Amen.

Three

What Are Your Motives?

Terry bubbles with excitement as she tells her friends about her new relationship with her mother-in-law. 'We've hated each other for years!' she explains. 'Now, what do you think has happened? She told my husband that since I've lost weight, the change in me has been miraculous!'

The other women nod their heads in understanding. 'And how do you feel about your mother-in-law now?'

'I feel closer to her, somehow. Maybe one day I'll really love her. She's so much nicer to me now.'

Terry realizes that the cause of the poor relationship was due more to herself than her mother-in-law. Over-eaters are often selfish people who look at self-denial as punishment rather than a healthy response to the love of God. Terry succeeded in losing 4st 6lb, and in the process, learned a great deal about herself. 'I never realized what a self-centred person I was!' she confessed. 'I ate out of anger, frustration and even jealousy. I blamed my problems on everyone else.' She realized that she hated sharing her husband with his mother and resented her role in their lives, something she would never have admitted to herself before.

If Terry's motives for losing weight had been selfish,

she would have fed one of the strong motives that caused her to overeat in the first place. That's why her previous attempts had always failed. She had been on dozens of diets before, and always regained the weight she had lost. This time she made a firm decision after she committed herself to the task of losing weight. Her decision to lose weight was to please the Lord.

We have as our ambition, whether at home or absent, to be pleasing to Him (2 Cor 5:9).

A motive is the reason why we behave in a certain way. As a Christian, our motives are to be based on the word of God. There are some strong words regarding motives in the Bible. If our motives are for earthly gains or rewards, we will not be pleasing to the Lord and therefore will not benefit by his blessings. Listen to what it says in Philippians 3:18 and 19:

For many walk, of whom I often told you, and now tell you even weeping, that they are enemies of the cross of Christ, whose end is destruction, whose god is their appetite, and whose glory is in their shame, who set their minds on earthly things.

And 2 Corinthians 5:10:

We must all appear before the judgment seat of Christ, that each one may be recompensed for his deeds in the body, according to what he has done, whether good or bad, [considering what his purpose and motive have been, and what he has achieved, been busy with and given himself and his attention to accomplishing] (brackets Amplified Bible).

These 'enemies of the cross of Christ' may not be heathens, but Christians. It's possible to be a Christian and still miss your own potential.

The Lord is saying the end is destruction when our god is our appetite, when our glory is our shame, when our minds are set on earthly things. He is not saying, 'If you want to eat a dozen doughnuts, go ahead. I understand. When you finish those, why don't you have some ice cream? Then you can fall on the sofa feeling sick and miserable, and watch TV.'

No, that's not the Lord. The Lord is telling you,

Delight yourself in Me. I shall fulfill the desires of thine heart (Ps 37:4 Author's paraphrase).

He is telling you to put aside all appearance of evil. He is saying, 'Cleave unto *me*.'

Did you know that you stifle God's work in your life when you habitually overeat? He is telling us that we're proud of things we should be ashamed of.

How many church buffets have you been to where you heaped your paper plate so high with food, you could hardly get it back to your seat without losing some of it on the way? How many times have you joked about who could eat the most?

Ask yourself this question: is it more pleasing to the Lord to exercise self-control or to eat anything, in whatever quantity I want?

'But I'm free from bondage!' you may protest. 'I'm free from the law. Jesus has set me free. Let no man be a judge of what I eat or don't eat. I'm free in Christ and I'll eat what I want. If I'm fat, so what? Jesus loves me and is not a respecter of persons.'

Now if that's what you're saying and believing, stay with us just a little bit longer. There are some real blessings in store for you. Self-control is not bondage; it's *freedom*. You are in charge of your life. Self-control is freedom! It frees you to be the real you.

● You use food. Food does not use you.

- You use calories. Calories do not use you.
- You are in control of what goes into your body.
- You are *free* from binging, gluttony and overeating.
- You are healthier, more energetic and in control of your life.
- You are no longer selfishly indulging in food.
- You are turning to God for your needs and desires to be fulfilled.

When your motives to please the Lord are clear and strong, you can be assured you will lose weight. God works from the inside out. Once your motives are in the proper place within your heart, you will begin to see results on the outside

> It is God who is at work in you . . . for His good pleasure (Phil 2:13).

Jesus did not come to earth to do any old thing he pleased. He came and lived in perfect obedience to his Father.

> And being found in appearance as a man, He humbled Himself by becoming obedient to the point of death, even death on a cross. Therefore also God highly exalted Him, and bestowed on Him the name which is above every name (Phil 2:8–9).

He became a model for us, showing us how to choose the right motivation.

> For it is God who is at work in you, both to will and to work for His good pleasure (Phil 2:13).

He wants to perform his perfect will in you and your life. He wants to fulfil his purpose for your life. You can lose pounds and be at the weight God intended you to be. Your motive is to please him. He's not punishing

you by taking food away from you. He is blessing you
and lovingly showing you how to walk in the power of
his Spirit.

Happily motivated

'Do all things without grumbling or disputing,' he tells
us, 'that you may prove yourselves to be blameless and
innocent, children of God above reproach in the midst
of a crooked and perverse generation, among whom
you appear as lights in the world' (Phil 2:14–15).

That's you and me—blameless and innocent and
above reproach in the midst of an overeating and junk-
food-eating generation!

Sometimes it's difficult to stop complaining about
the number of calories in a cream cake or how everything good to eat is fattening. But when our motives are
to please the Lord, we have the power within us to
rejoice in eating for his glory. This power is there waiting to be unleashed.

Our motives for losing weight in the past may have
been selfish. Maybe we wanted to be gorgeous for a
particular person or group of people.

Mary lost a stone for her school reunion. She wanted
to look smashing in front of all her old classmates. She
wanted to look as young as she did at school, and she
wanted to show up several of the other more popular
girls who were now fat and dowdy. Two months after
the reunion she had regained that stone plus an extra
5lb.

Do nothing from selfishness or empty conceit (Phil 2:3a).

There is nothing wrong with wanting to look attractive. God wants us to be attractive. In fact, when a
person becomes a Christian, he usually gains a new

attractiveness and vibrancy. The life within gives a glow and a radiance that wasn't there before.

The Holy Spirit gives new motivation to the Christian to be attractive. When selfish and vain motives creep in, the natural working of the Lord is hindered.

God wants to make you beautiful. He will help you be beautiful—if you let him.

PRAYER

Lord Jesus, I choose now to lose weight for your sake. I give up the old motives which have in the past failed. I choose now to eat to glorify you. I will lose weight to please you. Show me, Lord, what your will is for my body. In Jesus' name, Amen.

Four

Making Goals

Lois was always proud of the fact that she could eat whatever she wanted without gaining weight. Her friends ate salads while she ate rich desserts. They were the ones with the weight problems; she remained slim and trim. But one day she began to gain weight. Her clothes were too tight—zips bulged and buttons popped. She only had to lose a stone but it could have been a hundred. It meant disciplining her eating habits and this was as foreign to her as space travel.

Lois didn't wear her indulgences as some of her grossly overweight friends did, but she realized she had a problem that needed facing. 'I had never been aware that my overeating was a spiritual problem until I gained so much weight I couldn't fit into my clothes,' she told us at Overeaters Victorious.

'Now, with the Lord's help, I am learning how to eat. It is really hard for me because I'm just not accustomed to saying no to myself.'

In Lois' group there were women who needed to lose 4, 6, and 8st. Her stone seemed very little next to their extra weight. But Lois knew that if she didn't give the Lord control over her appetite now, her problem would only get worse.

How to find out how much you should weigh

How many times have you told yourself you want to lose so many pounds by such-and-such a day? How often have you said you want to weigh a certain weight because you used to weigh that?

Before determining your goals, stop and pray about it. Ask the Lord how much he wants you to weigh. Does that sound strange to you? One woman who had been on many diets in her lifetime and was still over-weight found asking the Lord how much she should weigh a phenomenon. 'I just never thought of it before,' she said. 'I prayed. I always prayed, but I just never thought of asking *him* how much *he* wanted me to weigh.'

When this woman did pray and ask the Lord to show her how much she should weigh, she found his answer to be different from her own plans. She had set herself high goals which she could never attain. On the few occasions she did reach the goals she set herself, she regained the weight within a short period of time.

'I always tried to get my weight down to 8st. But when I prayed, the Lord showed me he wanted me to weigh 9st. Well, that was a relief. I used to have dreadful fears about keeping my weight at 8st. I was afraid I'd have to starve to death to stay at that weight.'

How do you hear the Lord's voice? You ask and then you listen. It's amazing how many Christians have never heard the Lord speak to them. I don't mean in an audible voice. I mean hearing him deep within your own spirit. Ask the Lord how much you should weigh. When you're reasonably sure you have heard an answer from within your own spirit, pray about it. Then pray with Christian friends. It's important you pray with understanding friends, or friends who are also losing weight. Your mother or your wife or husband may not be the right one to consult. Your mother may love you podgy (she'd also love you if you had two heads and the plague) and your husband may say you're fine the way you are (he just has 'more to love', right?). Rubbish.

Ask people who are not personally involved with you. Ask them to pray with you. Tell them what you think the Lord is telling you and ask them how that sounds to their ears.

When a woman in one Overeaters Victorious group prayed about how much she should weigh, she heard the Lord telling her 8st 5lb. She was delighted to think she would one day weigh this. She asked her prayer partners to pray with her. Before they prayed, she told them the weight she thought the Lord was giving her as a goal. 'Oh, no,' said one friend. 'That's far too little. You don't want to weigh 8st 5lb. You'll be skin and bones.'

'You're large framed!' said the other. 'You'll need to weigh more than that.'

(Don't believe it if people tell you you're 'large framed'. Even if you're 8ft tall with very wide shoulders consider yourself average. One woman who lost 7st was shocked to discover she was actually a tiny person. You probably are too!)

'Are you *sure* it's the Lord who is saying that you should weigh only 8st 5lb?'

After more of the same discouraging discussion, the women prayed. After praying, each one told the woman she was right. The Lord told them the same. She is nearly at her goal as this book is being written.

So the first thing you do on your new weight-loss course is ask the Lord how much *he* wants you to weigh.

After you have asked this, you ask how many calories you should be eating a day in order to reach that goal.

Sometimes people aren't sure what it means to hear

the Lord speak. Here is an imaginary conversation between two Christians. One of them, a young man of 30, has recently lost 3st. His friend is a young woman who would *like* to lose 3st.

HE: I had the most wonderful experience in the cafeteria at lunch today.

SHE: Oh? What was that?

HE: I wanted to eat a fattening dish—it was spare-ribs soaked in greasy tomato sauce. Ugh! Anyway, just as I was about to order it, the Lord spoke to me and said, 'Don't eat that.'

SHE: What? What did you say?

HE: I said, I wanted to eat a fattening dish, spare-ribs soaked in—

SHE: No, no—I understood that part. It's the other part I didn't quite catch. *Who* said *what*?

HE: The *Lord* said, 'Don't eat that.'

SHE: That's what I thought you said. You're telling me that the Lord *speaks* to you?

HE: Yes, he certainly does. Especially about food, now that I'm committed to this new eating plan to lose weight.

SHE: You mean you hear voices?

HE: Not quite. It's not an audible *voice* I hear. It's like an inner knowing—

SHE: First sign of schizophrenia—hearing voices.

HE: I can assure you I'm no schizophrenic.

SHE: What sort of things does God say to you?

HE: He tells me how many calories I should eat each day in order to reach the weight he wants me to be. He tells me what I should be eating within that calorie limit.

SHE: The Lord tells you all that?

HE: Yes. He'd talk to you in the same way if you wanted him to.

SHE: But I'm no great saint or anything like that.

HE: Neither am I. I'm a simple believer. That makes me his child and he talks to his children.

(Pause. She looks long and incredulously at her slim friend.)

SHE: Does God actually go around *talking* to people?

HE: (Smiling.) He talks to his *own* people. I know that. His own people hear his voice and he knows them and they follow him.

SHE: Yes, I believe that. But how does he *talk* to you?

HE: It's an inner knowing. It's hearing his will through his voice deep within your soul.

SHE: In words?

HE: Yes, exactly.

SHE: What kind of voice does he have?

HE: He speaks through my own voice and my own thoughts. I'm the vessel he uses to speak to me. Naturally, he speaks through others and through his word, but he also speaks to me directly.

SHE: Is it something like having a conscience?

HE: Yes, it is. He will urge you not to sin and guide you into truth. But he says more. Your conscience doesn't tell you, 'I love you' or 'Well done, good and faithful servant.'

SHE: I'm a Christian and I believe that God directs my decisions. He guides me and helps me in everything. Why is this different from 'hearing his voice'?

HE: One is a bit more intimate than the other.

SHE: What can I do so that he talks to *me* too?

HE: Start by asking him questions and then listen for his answers.

SHE: Easy as that?

HE: You know, I read the book of Proverbs where it says, 'Hear the instruction of a father, and give attention that you may gain understanding,' and

I repeated those words. I said 'Lord, you have told
me right here in the fourth chapter of Proverbs to
hear instruction. Well, I'm listening. Please teach
me.'

SHE: But he does that through his word, the Bible.

HE: You're right, of course. That is our foundation
and it must always be the first word in all we do,
think, act and say.

SHE: I just can't imagine him telling me what to eat,
though. That seems so small, so insignificant.

HE: Eating is not an insignificant matter to me! Being
overweight has been a hassle for me most of my
life. It's affected my Christian life too. I've been a
compulsive eater, rebellious and self-willed. God
is now helping me change.

To many of us the idea of God speaking to us is
somehow far-fetched, weird or too good to be true.
He's only supposed to talk to a few select privileged
ones, certainly not *me*! When Neva Coyle was
interviewed by a reporter from the *Chicago Daily News*,
she happily told him, 'I ask the Lord what I'm supposed
to eat and he tells me.'

'Are you going to tell me that God *speaks* to you?' the
reporter asked with a slight sneer.

Neva answered, 'Are you going to tell me that water
goes over Niagara Falls?'

'I don't see what that has to do with my question,' the
reporter answered. 'Water going over a waterfall is a
natural event. A course of nature.'

Neva smiled and said, 'It's a natural event for God to
speak to us, too.'

'But surely he doesn't speak to just anybody!'

'But he does. God speaks to everybody. It's just that
many people don't listen.'

It is important on the OV weight-loss course that you

learn to hear the Lord speaking directly to you. However you hear his voice, whether it's an inner knowing, a direct word or a blast of trumpets in the night, you must get to know him and get to know what he's telling you.

Overeaters Victorious differs from other weight-loss courses. Most doctors and clinics will give you piles of papers with menus, diets, lists of can't have's and can have's. This gives you only one responsibility and that is to buy the food you're told to buy and eat it exclusive of all else. In effect, the overweight person becomes a servant of the weight-loss course.

This book won't tell you how many calories you are to eat and what you are to put on your plate at each meal. You get those instructions from your Lord. He's the One who wants to live in it with you. He loves you more than anybody else in the whole world and is more concerned with your weight than anyone else you know. Let him speak to you and direct every morsel you eat.

Please, if you're on a special diet ordered by your doctor for your health, or if you are taking special medication, do not change what you are doing without discussing it with your doctor.

A good 'test' of the word of the Lord, in fact, would be to check with your doctor and ask him if your calorie intake and goal weight sounds reasonable. The Lord isn't going to give you any instructions that are unwise, harmful to your health or unreasonable for you to accomplish. Your doctor's response should confirm this.

Hearing God's voice

This story was told by Jean, who had struggled with her weight for twenty-two years.

'Lunch time has always been the worst time of day for me. The kids are at school, my husband is at work and I'm alone. I can have really good intentions and put a cottage cheese salad on the table, but then something happens to me and I eat everything in sight. I'll stuff myself until dinner when I can hardly eat a thing. My husband wonders why I'm so fat when I don't eat anything. He doesn't see me stuffing myself all day. And he doesn't see me after everyone else has finished eating when I'm washing up.

'I've tried a lot of things, like getting the kids to wash up or getting out of the house during the day, but nothing lasts. I always go back to my old habits.'

After completing six sessions with OV, Jean wrote on her response sheet these glowing words:

'Early on when I was asking the Lord to speak to me, a wonderful thing happened. I had just finished a very *small* lunch of soup, salad and a sandwich (for me, that's small. I used to eat six sandwiches just as starters). I heard the Lord say to me, very clearly and distinctively, 'Now feast on me.'

'I got my Bible out and began to read immediately. Now every day I have lunch with my Bible open right in front of me so that when I finish the last bite, I begin to read the word. It works! You can see by my chart I've lost 10lb.'

Five months later, Jean was asked to share with others at an OV weekend retreat. 'I feel like a new person!' she bubbled. 'I've lost 2st 6lb and I've almost reached my goal. When God told me to feast on *him* instead of food, it was like a bomb exploding in my life. I have read more of the Bible and memorized more scripture in these past five months than I have in my entire fifteen years as a Christian.'

When the Lord speaks to you and you begin to obey his voice, you'll find yourself feeling and acting like a new person too.

Let your words and attitude be as the young boy Samuel's when the Lord gained his attention: 'Speak, Lord, for Thy servant is listening!' (1 Sam 3:1–18).

You are not alone in the battle against overeating. There are hundreds, even thousands, of others who are praying right now. And God is answering in their lives. He'll answer in yours. Don't be afraid to hope in God. In obedience to his word and his voice, your hopes of losing those pounds will become a reality.

Don't despair any longer. God is moving on your behalf. You *will* make it this time.

God promises success and prosperity in response to your obedience. Won't you take a moment to ask him to speak to you?

You *will* hear his will made clear to you if you listen carefully.

> And do not be conformed to this world, but be transformed by the renewing of your mind, that you may prove what the will of God is, that which is good and acceptable and perfect (Rom 12:2).

'Test the spirits,' the word tells us. So you can 'test' the word you receive by sharing it with others, carefully weighing it with the knowledge you have regarding nutrition and your own general health, and prayer.

If you think the Lord is telling you to go on a fad diet of, for example, only grapefruit and eggs for a certain time (or some equally unhealthy scheme), please pray again. God's ways aren't faddy—they're eternal and everlasting.

Your goal is not only to lose weight, but also to learn a fabulous lifetime pattern of new eating and living. You could eat sticks for a month and lose lots of weight, but you would also probably destroy your stomach. God doesn't want any part of you destroyed. He wants you beautifully built up and adorned in his Holy Spirit, powerful and lovely in his strength and glory.

PRAYER

Father, in the name of Jesus, I need specific guidance and direction in my life regarding my eating habits. You can see I need your help in losing the extra weight on my body. Show me your will. Please speak to me and show me how much weight you want me to lose, how much you want me to weight, and how many calories I need to eat each day. Speak, Lord, your servant is listening. In Jesus' name, Amen.

Five

On Your Way to a Slimmer You!

You have given your appetite and eating habits to the
Lord. You are on your way to an entirely new way of
eating and living. You are on your way to a slimmer
you!

> Do you not know that you are a temple of God, and that the
> Spirit of God dwells in you? (1 Cor 3:16).

The Lord Jesus and the word of God are directing
your motives for losing weight. You will not only lose
weight, you will also make your body (your temple)
stronger and healthier. What a wonderful temple for
the Holy Spirit to dwell in! A strong, firm and healthy
temple, not overfed, undernourished, flabby and sickly.

> If any man destroys the temple of God, God will destroy
> him, for the temple of God is holy, and that is what you are
> (1 Cor 3:17).

You will be feeding strength and vigour into your
body. Instead of the overfed and undernourished body
you've been accustomed to, you will be lighter, fresher
and more energetic.

One woman who was at least 3½st overweight, possibly more, tells how she was afraid to lose weight. 'I need the extra weight in case I become ill,' she said. If you have that notion anywhere in the back of your mind, you can remove it now. Being overweight hinders health; it does not help it.

At a conference on Obesity held at the National Institute of Health, biochemists, physicians, psychologists and sociologists came up with a number of findings that we all ought to be aware of.

1. Men under the age of 35 who have been fat all their lives seem to have a higher cardiovascular disease and diabetes risk.
2. A 15st, 35-year-old man who should weigh 11st raises his risk of dying suddenly by 67%.
3. Obesity in adulthood is associated with diabetes, heart disease, high blood pressure, gall bladder disease and cancer of the uterus.
4. Obese males have a high risk of sudden death. (Although the risk of dying prematurely is much greater for obese males than for obese females.)
5. Coronary heart disease would decrease by 35% if everyone were slim.

Dr William Kannel, director of a study on obesity, said, 'Except for stopping cigarette smoking, the correction of overweight is probably the most important thing that can be done to control cardiovascular disease.

'We need a greater sense of urgency about obesity,' Dr Kannel asserted. 'As we now do when a lump is discovered in the breast, something should be done immediately when a child is obese. This is a public health problem, not an individual doctor-patient problem.'

Edward Lew, an actuary for the American Cancer Society, said that men aged 35 who are 20% above the optimal weight level are likely to lose 5½ years of their lives.

The deep-rooted belief that fat means health is an inaccurate one. In days past, to be thin meant to be hungry. Weight loss was usually associated with sickness.

Change your thinking to *slim is healthy*.

We are not saying that you should be anorexic. No, you should be a fit vessel for the Master's use.

> And you shall know the truth, and the truth shall make you free (Jn 8:32).

If you think the Lord is telling you to eat fattening sweets for energy, you may need to do some more reading of the word. God does not starve his beloved children with sugary foods that do not nourish the body. He doesn't prescribe greasy, fattening foods that actually rob you of energy. As one woman aptly asked, 'If Jesus were here today, would you see him coming out of a supermarket with twelve packets of crisps, one for each disciple?'

When Jesus was preaching by the sea of Galilee, a great crowd of people were following him. They were excited and awed at the signs and wonders the Lord was performing. Sick people were being healed, the lame were walking; oh it was one of the most thrilling spectacles they had ever seen.

Then Jesus went up on a mountain and sat down with his disciples for a while. The Passover, the feast of the Jews, was at hand, and Jesus was concerned that the people needed to eat. As always, his concern was for the people.

He looked up and saw the hoards coming towards them. He knew they had been following him in the heat and dust, pressing together in the great crowds, and they were hungry.

'Philip, where are we going to buy bread that these may eat?'

Take note: the Lord did not say, 'Where are we going to buy Mars bars that these may get some quick energy?'

They didn't have enough money to buy bread for such a great host of people. Then Andrew told the Lord, 'There is a boy here who has five barley loaves and two fish.'

This pleased Jesus. 'Have the people sit down,' he said. They were going to have a feast. And the feast for this hungry and tired crowd was a high protein meal. Jesus took the loaves and thanked God for them. He distributed to those who were sitting down and then did the same with the fish. Everybody ate as much as they wanted and there were twelve baskets filled with left-over food. The Lord multiplied a nutritious meal for the people.

If it's energy you want eat protein, not sweets.

Your goal, remember, is to eat in obedience to God through the power of the Holy Spirit.

The Lord wants to help your walk of obedience. That help comes through being completely his. Your attitudes have to match his will for you. Your commitment to him has to be complete, your goals his goals, your attention given completely to obeying him, your obedience in his power.

You cannot fail when you give yourself completely to him.

> For those who are according to the flesh set their minds on the things of the flesh, but those who are according to the Spirit, the things of the Spirit (Rom 8:5).

You have prayed and given your eating habits to the Lord. You have given your life, your entire being to him. You are totally his, surrendered to him. Your desires, appetite, longings, dreams, ideas and thoughts are his. Your mind is set on the things of the Spirit.

> For the mind set on the flesh is death, but the mind set on the Spirit is life and peace (Rom 8:6).

You will no longer turn to food when you are frustrated, nervous, worried, feeling rejected and unloved, or bored and depressed. You will turn to the word of God, filling your mind with its power and wisdom and strength. Through concentrating on the word—meditating on it and being in constant communion with the Lord—you find life and peace.

> Because the mind set on the flesh is hostile toward God; for it does not subject itself to the law of God, for it is not even able to do so; and those who are in the flesh cannot please God (Rom 8:7–8).

Times of dieting in your own strength, or in the flesh, are past now. You receive God's blessings by knowing and doing his will for you. Now you are no longer deceived. You know God wants to help you lose weight. You know he loves and cares for your body and is right beside you helping and blessing you as you lose weight for his sake.

> However you are not in the flesh but in the Spirit, if indeed the Spirit of God dwells in you...the Spirit of Him who raised Jesus from the dead dwells in you, He who raised Christ Jesus from the dead will also give life to your mortal bodies through His Spirit who indwells you (Rom 8:9a, 11).

If the Spirit of God could raise Jesus Christ from the dead, he can surely help you lose weight! You have a great source of strength within you now. When you begin to tap its resources, you will soar with unreserved strength and power.

You are in control

Let no one act as your judge in regard to food or drink or in respect to a festival or a new moon or a Sabbath day— things which are a mere shadow of what is to come; but the substance belongs to Christ (Col 2:16–17).

This means that you are in control of your eating habits through the power of the Holy Spirit. Your best friend may say to you, 'Oh, go on, have a piece of pie. I baked it just for you!'

If your friend really loves you, she or he will respect your desire to please the Lord and lose weight. They'll understand when you refuse the pie.

Ann comes from a large Italian family who love to eat. The rich pastas and desserts had put an extra 6st on Ann's small frame. Going home is always a trial because her mother insists: 'have another helping', or 'eat your dessert—I baked it just for you!' Ann has had to be assertive with her mother and tell her point-blank, 'Mama, I am on a weight-loss course to please the Lord. I want to please him by my eating habits. That is why I am saying no to another helping of lasagne and I won't have a canoli.'

Her mother may be hurt, but it won't last. Feeding someone rich and fattening foods is some people's way of expressing love. If you show them that food does not mean love to you, they will learn to express their love in other ways.

Friends may tell you things like, 'You—lose weight? That's crazy. You're not fat!' or, 'Come on, it won't hurt to go off your course just this once!' It may be a temptation to listen to them and do as they suggest.

You do not have to give in to temptation! You can rise above it. You are living a *new* life of discipline and self-control. The food may be very tempting, but you don't have to eat it.

'No,' you answer, 'I will not eat that. Please don't ask me to fail.'

Diets that hurt

> Let no one keep defrauding you of your prize by delighting in self-abasement and the worship of the angels (Col 2:18a).

Dieting in the flesh leads to delighting in self-abasement. When you are losing weight for the Lord and with his help and encouragement, you will not degrade yourself or your body. The reason is, you are aware of his love for you. He cares deeply for you and for the health and vitality of your physical body. You are now eating to please him. You won't defile or hurt something that is precious to the Lord.

Your body is precious to the Lord. Here are some ways your body can be hurt. Avoid them!

Fad diets.

Diets which require your eating only one kind of food such as a grapefruit diet or a banana diet or an all-protein diet are harmful and dangerous to your body.

A young woman sat sullenly in an OV meeting, her eyes glazed, staring straight ahead at the leader. A woman sitting near her noticed her for two reasons. One was that she was definitely not overweight; in fact, she was underweight and looked gaunt and undernourished. Second she had a distant and faraway look in her eyes, as though she were in a mild daze.

After the meeting she asked to speak privately to the

group leader. She told her she had recently lost 4½st on predigested liquid protein. But she was suffering heart tissue damage and nervous disorders. Furthermore, she was afraid to eat. She had been fat all her life and was worried that she'd regain it all if she started eating again.

God does not hurt our bodies, damage our hearts and destroy our personalities when he blesses our weight-loss course. God does not fill us with fear or anxiety about eating. He gently teaches us how to eat properly so that we will never be overweight again.

Dr Philip White, director of nutrition for the American Medical Association, said more money is spent on 'worthless cures for obesity than for all medical research combined—and America grows fatter.

'Weight loss without rehabilitation of the lifestyle that allowed the person to gain is fruitless,' he said.

Fasting for weight loss.

Going without food at all can be just as drastic for the overweight person as binging. It is an extreme just as overeating is. If you are going to fast, please fast for the purpose of prayer and intercession, not to lose weight. You will regain the weight you lose and your efforts will have been in vain.

Some hospitals use the fasting method for the dangerously obese and gradually wean the person back onto a calorie-restricted diet. There will be a large weight loss to begin with and later the weight will be lost gradually.

Obviously you will lose weight on a fast, but it may not remain lost. Obese people can tolerate a prolonged fast better than slim people. During the early stages of fasting (first four to fourteen days) weight loss is substantial, but it is primarily water loss and easily regained.

Weight loss by fasting is greater in heavier people than lighter people. During the early stages of a fast, as much protein is lost as fat, which is not desirable. This loss may result in the stunting of hair growth and/or dry and scaly skin. As the fast progresses, fat loss increases more than protein loss.

There are some advantages to fasting, including giving the overworked internal organs and tissues of the body a good rest and time for rehabilitation. Fasting (over six days) flushes out toxic matter and poisons from the system. Fasting improves circulation and promotes endurance and stamina. Fasting renovates, revives and purifies the cells of the body.

Despite these advantages to fasting, do not do it for the purpose of losing weight. It is important to learn how to *eat*.

If you have died with Christ to the elementary principles of the world, why, as if you were living in the world, do you submit yourself to decrees, such as, 'Do not handle, do not taste, do not touch!' . . . These are matters which have, to be sure, the appearance of wisdom in self-made religion and self-abasement and severe treatment of the body, but are of no value against fleshly indulgence (Col 2:20, 21, 23).

Drugs, slimmers' foods, shots, surgery, etc.

These are not the real answer. The lasting way to lose weight and keep it off is to change your eating habits. In desperation to lose weight, some choose painful and dangerous by-pass surgery. In addition to the painful and tedious recovery, the surgery is effective for only five years. For some it doesn't last that long.

How did you get fat in the first place? Fleshly indulgence. How did you lose weight and regain it? Fleshly indulgence. How do you stay fat even though you want to be slim? Fleshly indulgence. Why do you gain weight instead of losing? Fleshly indulgence.

You can't cut fleshly indulgence out with a knife. You can't remove it with drugs before meals or a powdered drink instead of a meal. Eventually it will rear its head again.

Other weight-loss methods, including hypnotism, acupuncture and vomiting, will not produce lasting healthy results either. Such things 'are of no value against fleshly indulgence'.

> Let no one keep defrauding you of your prize by delighting in self-abasement (Col 2:18a).

The Lord is your judge and *you*, by the power of the Holy Spirit within you, control your responses to his directions. He will show you the foods you are to eat and how to eat them, if you will let him.

The Lord is encouraging you and giving you strength and power.

> ...He who began a good work in you will perfect it until the day of Christ Jesus (Phil 1:6).

He is not going to allow you to fail.'

But first you must forsake the fad diets and restrictive diets you have attempted in the past, confessing their total inadequacy against fleshly indulgence. These diets, devices and promises have had 'the outward appearance of wisdom, in self-made religion, and self-abasement and severe treatment of the body, but are of no value against fleshly indulgence.'

PRAYER

Dear Jesus, I repent of fleshly indulgence. I confess that I have attempted to lose weight in the past outside of your will. Forgive me, Lord, for not taking the strength and wisdom you so freely and readily give. I know you love me dearly, Lord, and for that reason I will not hurt or debase my body. I will bless my body in the name of Jesus.

I conquer fleshly indulgence in the name of Jesus Christ. I now begin a new way of eating and living according to the word of God and the power of the Holy Spirit. I turn from the old, useless ways to the new, bright and beautiful. My hope is in the Lord and not in diet.

I hereby refuse, in the holy name of Jesus Christ, to put my trust in fad diets, fasting, drugs, surgery or any other false promise. I declare myself free from these 'outward appearances of wisdom'.

I am now free to lose weight your way!

In Jesus' name, Amen.

Six

We Are Not Learning to Diet

Your days of dieting are over. You are now beginning a new way of *eating* and *living*, not dieting. You're on your way to health and slimness.

For some people 'calories' is a dirty word. They don't even want to hear that word. They hate the idea of calories and hate even more the idea of counting them. But you are going to count calories on your new weight-loss course. However, we use calories; they don't use us.

One OV group leader calls calories 'God's little helpers'. She tells her new members that 'God's little helpers' are for our benefit, not our dismay. Some people seem to feel that a calorie is an enemy. They are accustomed to thinking everything delicious is loaded with calories, and counting them would be a horrendous chore, not to mention discouraging.

The reason we don't advise everyone to go on the same diet of a certain fixed number of calories is that each body is different, and the aim is not to learn how to diet, but to learn how to *eat*.

Each individual is highly unique and important to the Lord. He loves each of our bodies and created them perfectly and specifically according to his perfect design and measurement. It is important for you to hear him give you his own calorie quota.

In one group of twenty-five people, for instance, there may be twenty-five different calorie quotas. One woman will be eating 1,000 calories a day, another 800, another 950, and so on. Pregnant and nursing women need more calories.

You count calories to be intelligently in touch with what you're putting into your mouth. You will become aware of those 'innocent' little nibbles. You'll be using calories for your benefit from now on. After the Lord tells you the amount you can have, you'll be planning and carefully working out the best ways to 'spend' them.

What is a calorie?

Energy available in food is expressed by calories. They provide the energy needed for us to breathe, digest food and maintain body heat in order to fulfil the body functions that comprise our metabolism, or basic life processes. Age lowers metabolism and that's why older people require fewer calories. You need calories to keep your body functioning and to supply you with the energy for muscular activity you do each day.

Excess calories are equal, no matter where they come from. Energy, whether coming from a piece of cake or a sirloin steak, is equal, in that energy not used by the body is stored in the form of fat.

The nutrient composition of cake and steak are not the same, however. Cake has little, if any, available nutrients. Steak contains protein, carbohydrate and fat. When counting calories don't consider a slice of cake and steak equally beneficial to your body simply because they may have the same amount of calories.

Overweight people often don't take time to learn

about nutrition. Perhaps they don't want to know that the foods they crave are bad for the body. One woman, so fat she could hardly sit in her chair, went to a lunch and ate the most fattening foods on the menu, telling herself and others, 'Oh, this isn't fattening. After all, everything in it is healthy. Meat, eggs, cream, butter—it's good for me!'

She couldn't be more wrong. The nutrients were minimal, but the calories were present in huge quantities.

Some nutritionists suggest cutting your calorie intake by a third to lose weight. That's okay if your doctor agrees, but you will want to use the calories you do eat to your advantage. Any person on a weight-loss course should eat protein. Protein feeds your appetite in the hypothalamus in your brain. It stops those urges and cravings for sweets and unhealthy foods. Be sure to spend the biggest portion of your calories on protein foods. Eat protein at every meal and you'll lose weight faster, have more energy and have better muscle tone than if you starved yourself on salads only.

Your daily power

Every morning have a time of Bible reading and communication with the Lord. This time of communication with him is important. A good place to begin reading is in the book of Colossians. From there you could read the other books of the New Testament, combined with the Psalms and Proverbs. Some people are addicted to drugs; you're addicted to the Lord. You must go to him for your supply of strength for the day and for your instructions. This is vital.

Every morning after you have had your time of reading the Scriptures and praying, ask the Lord what you should eat for the day according to the calorie allowance he has given you. Then in a notebook make a record of this.

Eat only what you have written down for the day and no more. If you do go over, be sure to enter it and the amount of calories. This is not meant to put you in bondage, but to introduce to you the joy of having *control* over what goes into your mouth.

When you see that those 6 nuts you nibbled before dinner cost you 100 calories, you will want to start controlling those urges to nibble.

Your notebook will become your diary. OV members treasure their diaries; some say they will keep them for life. You will be amazed at what you learn about yourself through your diary.

In your diary, on a separate page from the calorie sheet, write the verse you read for the day and what it means to you. Begin each entry with a verse of Scripture and then apply it to yourself, making it personal.

One woman's entry in her journal for the day read:

1 Samuel 15:22: 'Has the Lord as much delight in burnt offerings and sacrifices as in obeying the voice of the Lord? Behold, to obey is better than sacrifice, and to heed than the fat of rams.'

I've heard this scripture a million times, but somehow now it means more to me than ever before. I just never realized what it meant until now. I've lost two pounds this week and I am thrilled with the discipline the Lord is teaching me. How many times have I sacrificed the wrong things to the Lord and sacrificed for the wrong purpose!

I feel so happy to be obeying Him! I write down my calories every day and I think I'm really happier in being obedient than I am in the actual weight loss. It's wonderful! I have obeyed for two days straight and I feel happier than I've felt in months.

I'm really learning it's more important for me to obey the Lord than it is to lose the weight I'm losing. I love knowing I am obeying the Lord. I love feeling good about myself and I feel good about myself when I'm obedient.

There are some people who are against the idea of keeping a diary. Some of the excuses they might use are: somebody else might read it and discover their secrets, they don't have time, it's too much bother, and they don't have the privacy to do it.

Please don't allow these or any other excuses to rob you of the enormous benefits of keeping a diary. OV people carry their diaries with them during the day. Women carry them in their bags along with a small-sized Bible. Men can carry them in their jacket pockets, briefcases or lunch-boxes.

One woman said, 'I don't think I really knew myself at all until I began reading my own diary. I can't tell you what a revelation it has been. I'm discovering *me*!'

Fat people often dislike any kind of discipline. They often don't want to give up anything, don't want to lose anything; they often can't stand rejection, and they eat to compensate for the things they lack and failures in their lives.

You are now waging a war against overeating and being fat. You are waging a war against your own reasons for overeating. You will not be a fat person any longer when you start developing discipline and control in your life. You are fighting for the real you to emerge. That person is one who is *not* afraid of discipline. Because of this you should:

1. Be sure you don't miss your time of reading the word and praying early each day.
2. Enter on a separate page in your notebook the calories and food you will eat for the day.
3. Record in the diary your verse of scripture for the

day and what it means to you. Enter your thoughts, feelings and moods too.

Because your commitment to the Lord in losing weight is a real and wholehearted one, you *will* succeed.

Summary

Keep your diary up, trying not to miss a single day. This discipline is good for you! Think of it as an honour to do it unto the Lord.

Keep a record of calorie intake at each meal. Total your daily calories to be sure you are staying within the limit the Lord has given you.

Prayer and reading the word daily are as vital to you as breathing. You are dependent upon the Lord and his word to fill you and strengthen you every day.

You are gaining control over food. Food will no longer control you.

But thanks be to God that though you were slaves of sin, you became obedient from the heart to that form of teaching to which you were committed (Rom 6:17).

PRAYER

Thank you, Lord, for teaching me discipline. I thank you especially, Lord, that I am now free from being a slave to calories, and I can use them for my benefit. I choose to receive from you the strength I need to be faithful to my commitment to you about losing weight. I choose to receive from you the help and encouragement I need to faithfully write down the food I eat and its calorie content.

I thank you, Lord, that I am victorious in you.

I will read your word in the strength of the Holy Spirit.

I will record calories in the strength of the Holy Spirit.

I will pray in the strength of the Holy Spirit.

I will retrain my eating habits in the strength of the Holy Spirit.

I am victorious because you are victorious!

In Jesus' name, Amen.

Seven

Pass the Celery

You can burn up fat without wearing yourself out or almost starving yourself to death. You can eat fat-fighting foods. Many vegetables, for instance, are so low in calories that the metabolic process of digesting them requires more calories than are contained in the vegetable itself. Take celery for example. Approximately 25 calories of energy are needed to digest a cup of cooked celery or 2 stalks of raw celery. There are only 10 calories in the celery itself, so by eating 2 stalks of celery you've burned up 15 calories.

There are many fruits and vegetables that are fat-fighting foods. Some of them are: apples, green beans, beetroot, broccoli, sprouts, cabbage, carrots, cauliflower, cherries, cucumbers, grapefruit, grapes, lemons, lettuce, mushrooms, nectarines, onions, oranges, parsnips, pomegranate, raspberries, radishes, spinach, tangerines, strawberries, tomatoes, watermelon.

Your body will use more calories digesting fresh fruit, such as oranges, than if you drink only the juice.

These foods actually help you burn up body fat. They are rich in vitamins and minerals that form the fat-fighting enzymes.

Protein is also a fat-fighting food. Protein increases your metabolism so that you burn up 130–140 calories for each 113 calories of protein that you eat.

A mistake people make when losing weight is to cut out protein from their diet. A 'dieter' eats low-calorie foods, but may tend to ignore the importance of fat-burning and energy-building protein.

Your body needs protein at each meal to keep your body sugar level high and prevent hunger and over-eating. Your body needs protein to repair tissues and help wounds heal. Your body needs protein for skin, hair, nails, vital body chemicals, blood and all organs and soft tissues. If you eat protein at each meal, you will not be depriving your body of vitally needed energy.

Complete proteins are meat, fish, poultry, eggs, low-fat cheese, skimmed milk and yogurt. Additional protein foods are beans, lentils, seeds, nuts, whole grain cereals and breads. Three ounces of broiled chicken has 20g of protein and so does a cup of cooked split peas. But the chicken has 115 calories and the peas have 290.

You need to check in your calorie counter which proteins are lowest calorie-wise and what size portions to eat. One woman neglected to check her calorie counter for the number of calories in chicken. She thought she already knew without looking it up. She was unfortunately mistaken in thinking there were only 100 calories in half a chicken. She was eating two chickens a day and couldn't understand why she wasn't losing weight. She thought she was eating 400 calories in protein and she was actually eating 1,200! Combined with the rest of her calorie intake, she was eating more than she needed to maintain her goal weight.

Let your eyes look directly ahead, and let your gaze be fixed straight in front of you (Prov 4:25).

One male OV member said, 'Sometimes I feel as if I'm fighting an addiction, a physical addiction—as much as any kind of alcohol, tobacco or drug addiction. My only weapon is the word of God. I choose to stand on the word. The Lord says in his word he won't forsake or leave me.'

You have your goal set before you. You have purposed in your mind to succeed and you will. Be meticulous in counting your calories and planning the best way to spend your calorie quota.

Shopping

Before you go shopping, arm yourself with the word of God. Use these words as your weapon against fleshly indulgence:

> But put on the Lord Jesus Christ, and make no provision for the flesh in regard to its lusts (Rom 13:14).

Write those words at the top of your shopping list in bold letters: *make no provision for the flesh*. Carry them in your hand. Repeat them again and again to yourself.

You will absorb the power in those words and do your grocery shopping in the spirit instead of the flesh.

Make sure you go shopping *after* you've eaten. Do *not* go to the shops hungry. Your shopping list of high-protein and vitamin-mineral-packed foods is in your hand. You have your eyes set with a fixed purpose, your gaze is straight before you. You're not going to stop and linger in the cake area. *Too expensive!* You won't spend your precious calories on those items. In fact, you should skirt around all those areas that may be too tempting for you.

Be nice to yourself. Wheel your trolley along the aisles of food that God placed there just for you. The heaps of beautiful fresh vegetables and fruits, and the refrigerators filled with marvellous protein foods such as yogurt (plain, of course), cheeses and low-fat cottage cheese. Then fill the rest of your trolley with poultry, fish, eggs, meat, whole-grain cereals and breads, and you'll have a good supply of healthy, energy-building meals to bring home.

'But if I bought those type of foods, my family wouldn't eat!' you may protest. Your family loves their high-calorie, low-value junk food, you say.

So did you at one time. That's why you're overweight today. You have been eating the wrong foods and you have been feeding the same to your family.

Here is what Barbara wrote on an OV response sheet:

> In the past four months I have lost 35lb and I am now only 10lb away from my goal. My eating habits have drastically changed. I went from being a junk-foodaholic to a responsible and nutrition-conscious person. In spite of this, I still found myself buying the junk food for my family! The foods I just wouldn't touch for myself I fed to them. I was really convicted about this. I felt as if I was poisoning them. They ate heavy, rich foods, sweets, greasy chips and other junk foods. I had to repent to the Lord for feeding my family what I couldn't have. It was as if I was getting some kind of subliminal kick out of their eating what I wasn't allowed to! Now they're learning to like healthier foods!

Letter after letter arrives at the OV office from women who are discovering they are the major cause for their family's poor eating habits.

If you have a family addicted to junk foods, first of all, remember who bought most of those foods for them. Then repent, ask the Lord for forgiveness and the ability to slowly wean them onto a healthier diet. Start by making luscious fruit salads, broiled meats (skip the rich gravies and substitute natural juices) and fresh, steamed vegetables. Try making healthy fruit juice drinks. For snacks, try introducing nuts and seeds, cheese and crackers, yogurt, fresh fruit. And instead of the sugar-packed cereals in the morning, try feeding them a high-protein breakfast of eggs, whole-grain bread or toast or a whole-grain cereal with honey.

Becoming acquainted with the contents of your cupboards

You'll be asking the Lord three things on your new weight-loss course.

1. How much does he want me to weigh?
2. What is my calorie limit to maintain a consistent weight loss?
3. Is there food in my kitchen that shouldn't be there?

This last item requires some special discipline on your part. Most fat people have a lot of food stored in the house, so this task will take some time and effort.

You will need to go through your cupboards, taking out each can, box and packet, and reading the labels. The purpose of this is to learn what you are putting into your body and the bodies of your loved ones. Experience has proved that fat people do not read labels, nor are they aware of the content of the foods they put into their mouths. Taste is the only important thing.

But you are losing the old 'fat' ways. You are becoming healthier, slimmer and *smarter*.

Be wise as a serpent, the Bible tells us. 'Wise' means able to reason and think. When you pick up a box of cereal and see the the first item on the list of ingredients is sugar and there's also a list of preservatives and chemical additives, plus a heap of calories to each serving, stop and re-evaluate whether or not it is wise to eat it.

Diane divided all the food from her cupboards, putting food she could eat on one side, and on the other side the food she couldn't eat. Then in another place she piled the food she didn't want anybody to eat.

She did the same with the food in the refrigerator. She used her notebook to write lists of products that were nutritious as well as low in calories. The other members of her family were not on a weight-loss course so they could eat certain foods she could not. But she didn't want them eating the junk food that had filled her cupboards for so long. It would take some gradual and loving retraining on her part to wean her family off the rich, gooey desserts and the convenience foods loaded with preservatives and chemical additives.

'It was a real shock to me to discover what was actually inside those boxes and cans. I learned that I was more influenced by advertising and commercials than I was by the truth. If a commercial on TV said that a food was nutritious and healthy, I went out and bought it. If an advertisement in a magazine had a picture of someone suntanned, healthy, slim and smiling next to a food product that was really junk, I'd buy it because the advertisement made it look healthy. I didn't realize what I was doing.'

Diane was like thousands who listen to the advert on TV telling you that a certain product is good for you. She bought the product without reading the label or finding out the real truth.

One mother said, 'Sugar is addictive. I know that. I have read about refined sugar and I know that it is just like putting poison into our bodies. It is addictive and makes us want more. It makes my children either hyperactive or slow. It makes me retain liquid. It makes me fat and makes my teeth rot. I have to ask myself, "Can I wholly and honestly feed sugar-laden foods to my family?" I want to be victorious and wise. The responsibility is mine.'

You may not think you eat much sugar, but when you take a look at your cupboards and refrigerator, you'll be surprised at what you discover. There's sugar in pickles, mayonnaise, soups, jelly, canned fruits, most cereals and all salad dressings. Sugar is often labelled as 'carbohydrates' and this may confuse you, an unsuspecting buyer. You may also see the following words on labels. They mean *sugar*.

Dextrose is a chemical sugar, derived synthetically from starch.

Fructose is fruit sugar.

Maltose is malt sugar.

Lactose is milk sugar.

Sucrose is refined sugar, addictive.

Glucose is a sugar found in fruits and vegetables. It is blood sugar, an essential element in the human bloodstream. Don't confuse it with the sucrose. They are not the same. Glucose is important to your health.

The advertisements may tell you that sugar is '100% natural', but so is rattlesnake venom. Read your labels. Know what you're buying.

Don't plan for failure

Sue, after taking a look at her cupboards, learned that she had a habit of tucking certain fattening items away for future failures. In case there would be a day when she no longer wanted to stay on her weight-loss course there was something in the cupboard to fail with, something fattening and loaded with calories.

Don't plan for failure. Plan for success! If you *plan* to succeed, you *will* succeed.

Fill your cupboards and refrigerator with foods you *can* eat. If your family eats foods that you can't, keep them where you can't see them. Don't leave biscuits in see-through containers if they're tempting to you. Don't leave sweets around if you're tempted to eat them. Don't store the cake where you can see it (especially if it has already been cut. You may be tempted to 'shave off a thin slice'—and then miserably discover you've shaved off and eaten half the cake). Besides this, clear the table when you've finished eating so you don't eat up the leftovers.

Marge gained 5lb one week although she rigorously stuck to her diet. She realized that nibbling on the leftovers had to be the reason. The crisp end of the roast beef, a lick of the peanut butter off the knife, the cake crumbs from the tin, the last of the gravy in the dish, the leftover macaroni—'just a teensy taste'.

Those teensy tastes can be devastating. One tablespoon of jam has 50 calories; half a cup of potato salad is 175 calories; one large oatmeal biscuit is 100 calories. The extra nibbling you do through the day may add up to enough calories for two meals.

You are committed to losing weight and getting your body under submission to the Holy Spirit. You are making no provision for the flesh and its lusts. You are no longer a person who has no control over what foods go into your body.

By becoming acquainted with your cupboards, you will find out some interesting things about yourself, as well as learn more about the foods you buy. You may discover, as one woman shared in her group, that she had been buying chocolate and sweets 'for her children', but she would hide them in the back of the cupboard and eat them herself. Those high-calorie foods you think you're buying for your family, children or friends have a way of never getting past you.

Perhaps you're like the woman who buys boxes of cakes ('for the family', of course) and on the way home from the shops, in the car, she eats one and then she eats another. She feels guilty about bringing home the cakes with two missing, so she finishes the whole packet.

Or maybe you've had the same experience as the man who bought a block of ice cream 'for the family' and ate every spoonful himself.

Check your motives for buying foods. *Make no provision for the flesh*. If having ice cream in the freezer is a stumbling block for you, don't buy it.

> Let your eyes look directly ahead, and let your gaze be fixed straight in front of you (Prov 4:25).

Remember, your goal is to be slim for the glory of God.

After you have eliminated the junk foods and high-calorie foods from your kitchen and filled your shelves with plenty of healthy, fresh foods, and your cupboards with fresh vegetables and fruits, low-calorie and nutritious foods, you can stand back and take time to feel terrific. You can see you are really serious about your commitment. The fruit of your desire really *is* to please the Lord. Your desire really *is* to be slim and glorify him in your body. It isn't just talk. You are acting on your commitment! You are free to be slim!

Millions of books on losing weight are sold each year; there's a multi-million-dollar business in over-the-counter pills, powdered drinks, chewing gums, exercise devices and a host of other items promising a slimmer you. You can rejoice that you are doing more than reading a book or buying a lot of diet paraphernalia. You are acting on a commitment to the Lord.

You have become acquainted with your cupboards. You are changing your eating habits.

> Stand fast therefore in the liberty wherewith Christ hath made us free, and be not entangled again with the yoke of bondage (Gal 5:1 KJV).

You're not in bondage to food when you're in control of what you eat. Bondage is slavery. And a slave has to do everything his master tells him. The biscuits in the Tupperware container can beat against the lid and call your name if they want, but you're listening to the strengthening, guiding voice of the Lord. The bakers and ice cream parlour can appear so inviting, you can almost hear them shout 'come on and eat!' from across the street. But you're not their slave any longer. You're free. You can say NO. And at home there is nothing in your cupboards to hold you captive. You won't be prowling out of bed at 3 a.m. to eat some ugly fattening thing. You're free from that bondage. You're free to be healthy, slim and beautiful to the glory of God.

PRAYER

Dear Lord, thank you that I am free to be in control of what I eat. Show me, Lord, the mistaken thinking that has held me in bondage and made me fat. Show me, Lord, the deceptions that have caused me to overeat and harm my body. I choose to be free in you. I choose to be free from the bondage to food that has caused me to be fat.

I repent, in the name of Jesus, of the deceitful eating I have done in the past. I repent of deviously buying wrong foods and telling myself they were for someone else. I repent of eating these foods.

Thank you, Lord, for the strength and direction you constantly give me. Thank you, Lord, for your great love for me. In Jesus' name, Amen.

Eight

A Word to Add to Your Vocabulary

Daniel, a man of God in the Old Testament, was not without his problems. Right from the beginning, he needed to make some important choices about his lifestyle and eating habits. He knew how God instructed his people to eat and he was dedicated to his Jewish traditions. But in the first chapter of Daniel, when Jerusalem was besieged by the Babylonians, Daniel was one of the young men taken captive to serve in the court of the foreign King, Nebuchadnezzar.

This king wanted Israeli boys who were:

1. Good-looking
2. Intelligent in every branch of wisdom
3. Endowed with understanding and discerning knowledge
4. Possessed with the ability to serve in the King's court.

When these young men were taken to the court of the King, they were to be instructed in the literature and language of the Chaldeans for three years. They were to eat the King's choice food and drink the wine he drank. Then, at the end of their three-year education, these 'chosen' ones were to enter the King's personal service.

Have you ever considered yourself in training for the

King of king's personal service? Do you believe yourself to be of the 'chosen' for God's service?

In the New Testament, the apostle Peter writes to 'chosen ones' who are aliens in foreign places. These aliens 'who are chosen according to the foreknowledge of God the Father, by the sanctifying work of the Spirit' (1 Pet 1:1–2).

A Christian is an alien without going to a foreign land. We're aliens because our real home is in heaven. This is our earthly dwelling place until the day we arrive in heaven.

One woman, upon studying this verse, said, 'I'm an alien in my own body! I don't belong in this fat body! The real me ought to live in a thin body!'

The body is visible evidence of the fruit of self-control.

There's a little word in this scripture passage that overeaters don't like. It's *obedience*.

The Christian is a chosen alien, 'chosen according to the foreknowledge of God the Father, by the sanctifying work of the Spirit, that [we] may obey Jesus Christ and be sprinkled with His blood: May grace and peace be [ours] in fullest measure' (1 Pet 1:1–2).

We have been chosen so that we may *obey* Jesus Christ! Then it goes on to say, 'May grace and peace be yours in fullest measure.' You may wonder why that phrase comes after the word 'obey'.

When you are in obedience you have grace and peace *in fullest measure*! It's a dazzling thought.

That's the position Daniel was in. He saw all those rich, choice foods and wines of the King's and he simply said, 'No.' (How easy it is to form the word no with our lips, yet how difficult to say it when there are rich, fattening foods around.)

Daniel and his three friends were the only ones who refused the King's food and wine. Daniel made up his mind that he would not defile himself with the King's choice food or with the wine which he drank (Dan 1:8).

Have you ever thought that your overeating was defiling?

'Defile' means 'to make filthy or dirty; befoul'. It means 'to tarnish the luster of; render impure, corrupt'. Further definitions are 'to make unclean or unfit for ceremonial use; desecrate and to violate the chastity of'.

Think of the last time you binged on some rich or fattening food. By eating that food, you were actually making your body filthy, unclean, unfit, desecrated.

Alarming, isn't it?

Usually when we overeat, it's not our bodies we're thinking about. We're more intent on satisfying an emotional need. (More about causes of overeating in chapter 17.) When you sit down to dinner, do you think about your heart, lungs, blood pressure, or tissue and muscle needs? Probably not. You're thinking about how hungry you are and how good the food looks and smells. You couldn't care less about your vital organs or metabolism.

Smokers have a similar disregard for their bodies' needs. A male patient, aged 42, is in a hospital with cancer of the throat. It's painful and life-consuming. In spite of his body screaming for relief from cigarette smoke, he continues to puff on three packets a day. His doctor is frantic. 'If you don't stop smoking, you'll die!' he pleads. The man looks him straight in the eye and says, 'Then I'll die—but I'll die smoking.'

For those who are according to the flesh set their minds on the things of the flesh, but those who are according to the Spirit, the things of the Spirit (Rom 8:5).

Gaining control of the flesh

Your flesh, or selfish worldly mind, is something you can control. Uncontrolled, our flesh is wild, unruly; it kicks its heels, rears its head against anything in its way. It is selfish, unthinking, propelled by stupid, meaningless passions. Your flesh has nothing good about it *unless* it is under the dominating influence and power of the Holy Spirit.

If your fleshly mind is in control, you'll defile your body at every opportunity. If you're at a party and there are rich foods on the table, you'll gobble them up without a thought. You may even continue to eat when you get home. Then you may find yourself on a fully-fledged binge!

Your flesh is miserable, wretched; doesn't know how to make a single wise decision. It always acts against the will and beauty of God.

The only time the flesh is beautiful is when it is listening and obeying the word of God. 'For the mind set on the flesh is death, but the mind set on the Spirit is life and peace' (Rom 8:6).

One woman shared how she had read a book on dieting in one sitting and by the time she had finished the last chapter, she had eaten six bars of chocolate and drunk a bottle of diet coke.

Well, at least there were very few calories in the coke, you may think, but the unhealthy chemicals and additives made up for the missing calories.

If our bodies had voices, the first thing they'd probably say to us is, 'Stop putting that rubbish into me!' They do tell us this, in fact, not with words, but with fat, pain, disease, lack of strength and vitality, nervous disorders, headaches and sleeplessness.

One woman tells how she was killing herself with her eating habits. 'And all the time I was nagging my

husband about his smoking. We were both killing
ourselves—he with nicotine and me with a knife and
fork.'

Daniel was chosen to serve King Nebuchadnezzar.
You and I are chosen to serve the King of kings. Our old
fleshly ways may have hurt our bodies with our
undisciplined appetites, but now we choose *not* to
defile our bodies. We choose *not* to eat the foods of the
world, those foods our flesh defiles us with.

'Those who are in the flesh cannot please God' (Rom
8:8). The incongruous thing about some Christians is
that in church they'll worship God in spirit and truth,
then after church they'll rush home and have dinner in
the flesh, wolfing down all sorts of defiling foods. It
seems odd to be in the spirit one minute and then, as
soon as food is brought into the picture, we abandon
our spiritual mind and jump right into the ways of the
flesh.

> ...the mind set on the flesh is hostile toward God; for it
> does not subject itself to the law of God, for it is not even
> able to do so (Rom 8:7).

Daniel did not abandon his spiritual mind. He
refused to defile himself with the King's food, and he
convinced the commander of the officials to allow him
and his friends to eat vegetables and water for ten days.
He told the overseer to see for himself at the end of the
ten days if they were not healthier and more robust
than all the youths who had been eating the King's
choice food.

Naturally, they were healthier and more robust than
all the others. So the overseer agreed to continue with-
holding the King's choice food and wine so they could
stay on their diet. Notice, Daniel wanted to *stay* on the
diet.

He wasn't doing penance by eating only vegetables and drinking water, or doing a short-term slim-up course. He *wanted* to eat that way. He didn't consider the King's choice food to be desirable at all. He found those foods distasteful and repugnant.

What do you think of when you say the word delicious? If you think of some rich, fattening thing, *stop*. You can change your ways of thinking. No longer consider King Nebuchadnezzar's choice food as delicious. Think of those rich, fattening foods as ugly, undesirable.

Food is not meant to tantalize and torment us. Food is meant to bless us and strengthen us. It is meant to satisfy our bodily needs for nourishment. Stuffing ourselves with fattening dainties to satisfy taste buds will never satisfy the tiniest spot of fleshly appetite. Fleshly appetite always calls out hungrily, 'More! More!'

You can train your mind to stop thinking of food as delicious, tantalizing, luscious, mouth-watering or any other such adjectives as long as you set your mind on losing weight. After committing yourself to Jesus instead of overeating, you must train your mind to think about winning the battle with food.

When a footballer goes into a game, he's all psyched up to win. The manager talks WIN, the crowds in the stands shout and cheer.

What do you tell yourself when you're out on the field fighting against fat? 'I'm going to WIN'? Or do you tell yourself fleshly words like 'Oh, poor me. Everybody else gets pie. I get carrots'?

There's tremendous power in your mind. God has given it to you. You have a strong will. Your will can choose the flesh or the spirit. You can blame Satan all you want for your fat, but he doesn't eat the food; you do. Satan may tempt you, but you're still the one who does the eating.

It's your flesh Satan appeals to. That is why it is vitally important that you reclaim your fleshly mind from his influence and put it where it belongs—under the power and influence of the Holy Spirit of God who loves you.

King Nebuchadnezzar talked with the young men and out of all the youths he had recruited, none was found like Daniel and his friends. When Daniel ate according to the wisdom of the Holy Spirit, he was rewarded not only with good looks and a healthy body, but also God's blessing of knowledge and intelligence in every branch of literature and wisdom, and understanding of all kinds of visions and dreams.

He and his three friends were ushered into the King's royal service and, once in, they proved valuable to King Nebuchadnezzar. When the King consulted them regarding matters of wisdom and understanding, he found them ten times better than all the magicians and conjurers who were in all his realm.

Their vegetarian diet was not the only reason for these young Jews' tremendous godly power, of course. Clearly, they prospered because they *obeyed* God. The diet was just the means God used to draw them into the intimacy with him that only obedience brings!

Look at rich unhealthy foods not as fattening, but as defiling. One girl said that she couldn't eat something if she found a hair in it. No matter how hungry she was, if there had been a hair in it, she couldn't touch it. Another woman felt the same way about flies, or other insects. If she were ever to find one in the food, to her it was defiled.

A woman once baked a layer cake in her oven. When the cake was cooked she opened the oven door and found a dead, cooked rat stretched across and stuck in the cake. Unknown to her, there had been a rat in the oven when she put the cake in to bake. Would you say that cake was defiled?

You wouldn't want to eat a hair, a fly, or a rat, but that eclair or those greasy french fries may be just as defiling. If you are disobeying God and eating more calories than you should be, cry out to the Lord for help. He won't turn his back on you. He is right there with you to help you. And don't ever give up. No matter how many times you stumble, get up and begin again. God loves you and doesn't give up on you.

> For I am confident of this very thing, that He who began a good work in you will perfect it until the day of Christ Jesus (Phil 1:6).

He's not going to forsake you in your hour of need. And if you stumble a little, he's not going to throw his hands in the air and give up on you. God granted Daniel favour and compassion (Dan 1:9) when he chose to eat vegetables and water for the glory of the Lord. He'll grant you favour and compassion, too, with your new eating plans because he loves you just as much as he loved Daniel.

PRAYER

Thank you, Lord Jesus, for favour and compassion in my eating habits. I have committed my eating to you, Lord, and I am committed to losing weight. I will obey you, Lord, and eat as you show me. Give me wisdom and knowledge so that I can be a blessing to others and to you.

I choose not to defile myself, as Daniel chose not to defile himself with ungodly food. I need your help and your strength, Lord. My flesh is weak. In the flesh I choose wrong things and I do not please you. But my mind set on the Spirit is life and peace. My mind set on the Spirit is *obedience* and a new body with which to praise you.

In Jesus' name, Amen.

Nine

Delighted and Fulfilled

Debbie woke up Sunday morning feeling very sorry for herself. She had arranged to go out to dinner with friends after church and she knew she'd have to eat a salad while her friends would be chomping away on the fattening foods she used to adore.

At church, she asked her pastor, 'When will this all end? Will I always be on a diet?'

'But you're not on a diet,' he responded quickly; 'you're learning how to *eat*, remember?'

'Yes, yes, but sometimes I feel like I'm on a diet. And it feels like I'll be on one for ever and ever.'

The pastor smiled at her and said, 'You know when the word tells us that "he who began a good work in you will perform it until the day of Christ Jesus", it means he'll keep working for a long, long time.'

Debbie was reminded that her new way of eating was not just something to do until she peeled off the weight she wanted to lose—it was *for ever*. Daniel didn't eat vegetables and water for ten days only and then binge on the King's food on the eleventh day.

You are going to have to eat the Lord's way, getting your body slim and staying slim—or you'll go back to the old ways of the flesh. You remember all too well those diet failures. You lost weight, reached your goal and then regained it all.

Debbie needed to discover *joy* in her new eating habits. She was devoted to losing weight and did everything right, but she needed joy in her life.

She didn't defile her body with wrong foods.

She wrote in her diary every day.

She stuck to the calorie allowance the Lord gave her.

She carefully went through her cupboards and removed every fattening and unhealthy food from them.

She steadily lost weight and on weeks when she didn't lose anything, she continued steadfastly in spite of discouragement.

But she lacked one thing: joy. Every meal was a trial for her. She watched her friends eat whatever they pleased. They were slim and she was fat. She saw the commercials on TV for rich and fattening foods, and her mouth watered. She saw the ads in magazines and on billboards and everything in her cried, 'I want!'

This can be one of the subtle pitfalls for the overeater. Some people go on a fast and spend more time in the kitchen than when they're not fasting. They don't eat, but they touch, feel, handle and prepare food. Their delight in food is still there, even though they're abstaining. One woman prepared a picnic dinner for her family while fasting. She prepared a huge bowl of potato salad, something she always loved to eat, and several other dishes. She was very proud of herself for preparing one of the most elaborate meals they had ever taken on a picnic.

She didn't eat one morsel. Her husband marvelled at her self-control and discipline.

When her days of fasting had finished, do you know what she did? She made a huge bowl of potato salad and ate the entire thing herself. It nearly killed her. She had to go to hospital and have her stomach pumped out.

It's important that we don't take inordinate *delight* in food. Did you know you can delight in it when you're not even eating it? Don't describe rich and fattening foods as 'yummy' or 'delicious' or 'out of this world'. They're not.

> Delight yourself in the Lord; and He will give you the desires of your heart (Ps 37:4).

He is our delight. Food is not our delight.

Overeaters Victorious delight in eating God's food, in obeying him and loving him. Our desire is to please him. Our desire is to love him and serve him with our bodies, souls and minds.

Are you asking God to take away an ungodly appetite? If you are, be sure you are not delighting in ungodly *thoughts* about food.

Don't crave for ungodly foods even though you're not eating them. The Lord spoke against wrong thoughts when he said that not only committing adultery was a sin, but thinking lustful thoughts was just as sinful.

> But I say to you, that everyone who looks on a woman to lust for her has committed adultery with her already in his heart (Mt 5:28).

When you ask God to take away your ungodly appetite, he replaces it with knowledge and intelligence in the matters of food and nutrition. If you're abstaining from ugly fattening foods but still drooling over them, stop immediately and change that way of thinking. Your delight is in the Lord and in thinking his thoughts!

Communication with God includes the attitude of your heart as well as your words in prayer. You communicate with him by your obedience (or disobedience) to him. You communicate with God by the attention (or lack of attention) you give him. God is approachable on levels other than verbal ones. Delight yourself in the Lord and your whole being will adore him. Your whole being is then fulfilled.

'Delight yourself in the Lord and He will give you the desires of your heart.' Who gives us our desires when we are submitted to God? God himself. It was he who gave you the desire to be slim. Your desire is *his* desire and your delight is in him.

Debbie had her *desire* in the right place—that is, she desired to please the Lord. She desired to change her eating habits and eat unto the Lord, but she didn't have any *delight* in it.

Delight means a 'high degree of pleasure or enjoyment; joy; rapture; great pleasure and satisfaction; to please highly'.

Debbie wanted to know how to delight in the Lord with her eating. She meditated on Psalm 37:4 and the following week told her group she was learning that she had only partially been obeying the Lord. She had followed her calorie allowances perfectly, but she did it with a resentful heart.

'Do all things without grumbling or disputing' (Phil 2:14) was the Bible verse she had written in her diary. 'When I was young, my father was very strict with me. He was always saying no to this or that. I couldn't do the things the other kids did or go places with them. I always obeyed him, but I resented his rules. I felt deprived.

'Now I see that I was behaving in the same way with the Lord. I would do what he told me to do, but I'd have no delight in it or in him. Losing weight was just like being deprived of the good, fun things again.'

Debbie is seeing how deceived she was. She is now

learning to *delight* herself in the Lord and obey him. She sees that it's Satan who deprives us by suggesting that ugly foods are delicious and we can't have them. He influences the flesh to eat ungodly foods and consider them mouth-watering and tasty. God gives, restores, lifts up, builds, strengthens and blesses. Satan destroys, kills, murders, lies, deceives. God is all truth and love. Satan has no truth or love in him.

Do you know what your own true desires are? The verse we are looking at in the Psalms reads, 'He will give you the desires of your heart.' Is it your desire to be slim? If it is, then ask yourself another question: 'Am I doing all I can to co-operate with God so that he can fulfil my heart's desire to be slim?'

If your desire is to be a certain weight, you will want to co-operate with the Lord so that you don't get in the way of his fulfilling your desire. OV members keep a Desire-Action Sheet such as the one below. You can make one for yourself. Write the desire of your heart that you are asking the Lord to fulfil. Opposite, write how you are co-operating with him to fulfil this desire.

Delight in your new way of eating. Delight in your commitment to the Lord. Delight in your calorie allowance. Delight in self-control and obedience to the Lord!

DESIRE	ACTION
1. I desire to weigh 8st	1. I will stay within the calorie limit the Lord gives me.
	a. By feeding on the word to bridge the gap between calories I eat and calories I want.
	b. Planning what I eat ahead of time.
	c. Making sure I have satisfying food in the house to eat.
	d. Being a wise shopper.

2. I desire to lose 2st in the name of Jesus and for the glory of God.

2. Keeping my diary, so as to be in touch with myself and observe pattterns and habits God is changing and breaking.

Barbara said that although she has lost 4st as an Overeater Victorious, her real joy was not in the weight loss, but in her obedience. 'I really *delight* in the Lord,' she told a group of new members. 'I have to tell you that through losing this weight, what the Lord did in my heart and life is far greater than the weight loss. I am new through and through.'

Delight yourself in counting calories. It is not drudgery or a hindrance! It is your freedom and your blessing. Thank God you can lose weight for Jesus! Thank God he is fulfilling the desires of your heart because your desires are his desires. That's how close you are to him. You are special and dear to him. You eat in the Spirit now, not in the flesh.

Make a Desire-Action Sheet for each week. What can I do this week? Keep it in your diary and refer to it as the week progresses. The reason for this is that you could write on the desire side, 'To lose 10lb,' and then a year later, you're still 10lb overweight. Your desires *work together* with your actions to produce results. Write your weekly weight-loss desire. Example: 'Lord, this week it is my desire to lose 3lb.' Then ask him how you should co-operate with him on this.

On the 'action' side of the paper you might write, 'Be faithful every day.' Well, you can't be faithful without the Lord. You need a daily 'power time'—a time of quiet before the Lord when you draw strength. You may want to subtract calories and add some prayer and Bible-reading time.

One woman wrote as a desire, 'To spend more time with the Lord.' As an action she had to decide just how she was going to do that, and she had to be specific.

The Lord wants us to be specific. Vagueness never brings specific results.

As her action she wrote: 'In order to spend more time with the Lord, I will turn off the TV in the afternoon. I will get up half an hour earlier in the morning and pray and read the word. I'll allow myself time every night before going to bed to pray and read the word.'

What would *your* specific actions be?

Diane was puzzled with her Desire-Action Sheet. She didn't honestly know what she wanted herself. She wondered, 'What are my desires?' She knew her mother's desires for her, she knew her husband's desires for her, and her children's, but she wasn't sure of her own.

On her way to a seminar of Christian works, she had hoped to fill out her Desire-Action Sheet on the plane. But she couldn't think of any desire *she* had. She knew her husband wanted her to lose weight, but she truly didn't know if *she* wanted to.

When she arrived at the seminar, she stood in a crowd of people and a complete stranger turned to her and said, 'Excuse me. I hope you don't mind my approaching you like this, but the Lord was just talking to me about you. He told me that you do not know the desires of your own heart.'

Diane gasped.

'But do you know what the Lord is also telling me?' he continued. 'He knows those deep hidden desires you have. It is his great pleasure to reveal to you those deep desires and he wants to fulfil them for you one by one. He needs your attention to show you, though.'

It was an experience that was to change Diane's life. She realized she had been afraid to think thoughts for herself or to be in charge of her own life. She began to pray boldly, seeking the Lord for herself and her own walk with the Lord. It wasn't too many days later when she was filling in the desire side of her sheet. And little by little, one by one, she saw these fulfilled.

Saying one thing—doing another

One good result the Desire-Action Sheet has is revealing the inconsistencies in our words. Often we talk about obeying, but we blatantly disobey. We'll pray, 'Oh, Lord, I just want to be your obedient servant. I want to delight in you with my heart and soul,' and then we'll run to the refrigerator for some high-calorie 'treat'.

The Lord doesn't reward us with ugly high-calorie 'treats'. He rewards us with power and strength in the Holy Ghost.

We say one thing, but mean another. We may say, 'I want to obey you, Lord,' on one side of the Desire-Action Sheet, and then go over our calorie allowance by eating a plateful of crackers and cream cheese.

We may discover we are a lot more rebellious than we ever dreamed. Thank God, he can change all that and save us from the bondage of rebellion. He is Saviour. He saves us from ourselves.

We are learning to say one thing and, at last, do the same.

PRAYER

Lord, I'm not going to just say you're Lord of my life. I'm going to behave and *act* as if you're Lord of my life. I'm going to declare you as Lord in all my actions.

I give you the right to tell me when to get up in the morning, when to go to bed at night, what to eat and what not to eat. I delight in you and I am going to act like it. In Jesus' name, Amen.

Ten

Who's Rebellious? Not Me!

Sandy insisted that she was large-framed and that's why she weighed so much. Her college friends agreed with her. (It was easier than arguing.) The truth was, Sandy had 17st on her medium-sized frame. She was plainly obese.

'For He Himself [The Lord] knows our frame' reads Psalm 103:14. We may tell ourselves we're not fat, we're only large-boned, but the Lord knows our frame.

Actor and college instructor, Richard Weed, was approached one day by a student asking to see his grade in an exam.

'What? You mean I only got a "C" in that exam?'

'Yes. That's what you earned. What would you rather have? An "A"? A "B"?'

'Well, I don't know—'

Richard handed him his pen. 'Why don't you put the grade you would prefer in the book. Here, go ahead. Do you want an "A"?'

The boy was speechless.

Then the wise teacher said, 'I'll do it for you. I'll erase the "C" and write an "A" in its place.'

When he had finished he studied the surprised

student. 'Tell me,' he said, 'do you know the material any better now?'

We are what we are no matter what lies we may tell ourselves. We may want to give ourselves "A's" when we only deserve "C's", and conversely, we may down-grade ourselves. (That's equally deceitful.)

Lack of honesty is a symptom of rebellion. If you can be dishonest in a small thing, you can eventually be dishonest in something big. That something bit is your honesty with the Lord. You promise to stick to a certain number of calories, but you rebel and binge. Or you promise the Lord to live for him and his ways, and you rebel and go your own fleshly ways. The Lord wants to save us from the deceitfulness of fleshly ways and give us beautiful, wholesome and complete lives in him.

Isaiah 30:1 says:

> Woe to the rebellious children, declares the Lord.
> Who execute a plan, but not Mine,
> And make an alliance, but not of My Spirit,
> In order to add sin to sin.

What is your most difficult problem with rebellion concerning food? Look at the following check list. Do any of these rebellious statements fit you?

- I eat without thinking about what I'm eating or how it may defile my body. After I've eaten I feel repentant and remorseful.
- I don't have any pleasures in life except eating. I don't want to give that up too.
- I want my chocolate (or whatever). It's not fair that I can't eat it when I want to.
- It's not my fault that I have a weight problem. It's my mother's fault. She's the one who got me fat in the first place. Now I can't help myself.

- God knows the pressures and problems I have in my life and that I eat because of them. Why doesn't God remove them if he wants me to be slim?
- I asked God to take away my appetite and he didn't so he must want me fat.
- If my husband didn't like to eat a lot of fattening foods, I wouldn't be fat.
- If my wife didn't cook such fattening foods, I wouldn't be fat.
- I come from a family of overweight people. That's why I'm overweight.

Add your own statements to the list. You see how dishonest rebellion is? The truth is, nobody else is the cause for your being overweight. Other people and factors may be the stimuli that trigger your overeating response, but the only one responsible for your overweight is you.

God wants to take the rebelliousness out of us. He wants to free us from that bondage which is worse than being in any prison. Whom the Son sets free is free indeed!

God waits for you to be willing to give up rebellious thoughts and actions.

Therefore the Lord longs to be gracious to you,
And therefore He waits on high to have compassion on you.
For the Lord is a God of justice;
How blessed are all those who long for Him (Is 30:18).

Not long ago we received a letter from a man who had lost 6st in prison. He had been in prison fourteen years and was almost 6st overweight. Have you ever complained that you couldn't change your eating habits because 'the conditions weren't right'?

Did you ever tell the Lord you couldn't possibly lose weight when you have a wedding, a luncheon, a party or Christmas just around the corner? The *conditions* aren't right.

This man found Jesus in prison. Eating prison food, unable to choose his own menus, he went from 18st to 12st. His words were, 'I made up my mind not to defile a temple of the Holy Spirit.'

If you don't think you can possibly lose weight in your present situation, you are mistaken. You *can* do it. God will show you how if you will let him. Take time to listen to him speak to you. He speaks to you through his word and in that still small voice within you.

> He, your Teacher, will no longer hide Himself, but your eyes will behold your Teacher. And your ears will hear a word behind you, 'This is the way, walk in it,' whenever you turn to the right or to the left (Is 30:20–21).

Every speck of rebellion has to leave you. Don't be afraid of the removal process. It's for your own good.

There are two things we can help the Lord with as he removes our rebellion. Firstly, by being willing to admit we are rebellious. If you don't think there's a shred of rebellion in you, then you won't know what's happening to you as the Lord tries to remove it. You'll get angry with him, yourself and anyone else around for getting in the way of *your* wants and demands.

Some people do not want to admit they are rebellious, especially overweight people. A woman overweight by at least 4st says defensively, 'I like to eat! God knows I like to eat. He made me this way, after all. If he wanted me slim, he should have made me a person without an appetite.' In effect, the woman was blaming God. And if she could blame God for her own overeating, she could blame him for any number of other things in her life. She could blame him for being ill, for running out of petrol on a deserted road, for her son's lost gloves, for her husband's lack of enthusiasm for the gospel, for her daughter's broken marriage, for the death of a parent.... In fact she could blame God for everything that ever went wrong in her life.

You must understand that putting the blame on God for such things is not biblical. It is anti-God. The Bible overflows with instructions to love him through thick and thin, to praise him, worship him, rejoice in him, love his word and his promises, be comforted in him, rest in him, believe in him, trust him.

It is not only ridiculous to blame God for your calamities and sorrows (including weight); it is wrong. Many of the events in our lives we call tragedies are not tragedies at all. They are really God showing his best for us by giving us a portion of his love far surpassing anything that went before.

'I'm *not* rebellious. God knows how I've suffered in my life. In spite of all I've been through, I'm still a Christian, after all.' These words come from the mouth of a rebellious person.

'I'm not rebellious,' are usually the words of a rebellious person.

When God removes rebellion, the process sometimes stings a little. You want your own way and he wants his. He wants to win over your selfish ways in order that you may be the winner.

He understands how we hate to let go of our stubbornness. That's why the Holy Spirit inspired these words in Proverbs 3:11–12, which he again repeated in the New Testament in Hebrews 12.

Despise not the chastening of the Lord; neither be weary of his correction: for whom the Lord loveth he correcteth;

even as a father the son in whom he delighteth (Prov 3:11–12 AV)

We delight him, therefore he corrects us! If your own father didn't delight in you, you now have a heavenly Father who does. It's a wonderful truth to think about and, if you will think about it with your whole mind, you will find it much easier to give up rebellious eating habits.

Eleven

Why Are We Attracted to the Wrong Foods?

Have you ever noticed that when you overeat, you don't do it with something like carrots or watercress? When is the last time you *craved* a stick of celery?

Did you ever binge on lettuce?

Your fleshly indulgences are usually something fattening, most likely something sweet, like dessert.

Whenever Barbara had a problem as a teenager, her mother would sit down at the kitchen table with her, bring out the chocolate cake and they'd talk over Barbara's problem while eating this and other high-calorie non-spiritual comforters.

Bev remembers when she was sad or upset as a young girl, her mother offered sweets to help her 'feel a little better'. If she came home from school upset about something a friend had said or done, her mother cut her a piece of something fattening, poured her a glass of milk, and said, 'You'll feel better after you eat this.'

Others share how, as children, they cleaned their plates in order to 'earn' dessert. Dessert, for them, became far more important than the meal. Later, when they really wanted to treat themselves, they chose dessert. And they're still choosing dessert.

Are you a chubby member of past Clean Plate Clubs

who gobbled up all the food on your plate, even though you were already at bursting point? You did it for the sake of the promise of things to come from the kitchen—luscious and tantalizing—*dessert*. You even gulped down sprouts and broad beans for the glorious reward of dessert.

Was that you cleaning up every scrap on your plate, choking on those last forkfuls of liver because over there, just beyond your reach, were better things.

Nothing was too dear a price to pay for trifle or cheesecake, or a similar mess.

Did you, at the age of 10 completely wipe out the hunger problem of India by eating every morsel of food on your own plate? Of course you did. You deserved a reward for that, you say. Your reward was dessert.

For all your consideration towards the millions of starving people of the world, you were rewarded with a fat body and bad habits. And India is still starving.

Then, later, was that you in line at the school cafeteria, passing right by the vegetables and salads, heading directly for the desserts?

And how about recently? Wasn't that you, when you were feeling a little blue, comforting yourself with a rich and calorie-loaded dessert?

The unconscious desire is to reward suffering. Desserts can become that reward.

If you are normally healthy (not diabetic or hypoglycemic) and you crave sweets, it may not be sweets you crave at all. Maybe it's energy you need. Sugar raises the blood sugar level in the body and some people get an energy boost after eating it. It's temporary, of course, and after the boost drops, you feel worse than before. So you eat more sugar.

Some Christians walk around droopy, tired and exhausted all the time. If you ask them, 'What's the matter?' they sigh, shrug their shoulders and tell you how tired they are. Worn out.

Sometimes the reason we feel like this is because we are taking into our own hands what the Lord wants to do. We get worn out in the flesh because we're behaving in the flesh.

There are times we get tired because our bodies are made of flesh, and when they are worked too hard or don't get enough rest, they get tired. It is okay to be tired *sometimes*. A football player may be tired after practice; a coach driver may be tired after a long run across the country and back; a teacher may be tired after an evening of marking essays. These examples are not due to anxiety-tiredness. Things that cause this sort of tiredness include: feeling nervous, or feeling frightened.

The Holy Spirit doesn't drive you, push you, force you, or overwork you. He doesn't give you so much work that you can hardly finish it without falling to pieces. Let go of your drives and let him work through you, accomplishing what he desires.

If you're craving an energy boost, your true source of power and strength is waiting for you. The word of God 'rejoices the heart'. Absorb and apply the truths and power in the word to your life. Allow its energy to permeate your being and see how unappealing a piece of chocolate or a sweet will seem to you.

When you are not in the word, you're not receiving your power pack of strength and vitality. Your spirit and soul are not fed on the true source of energy. Caffeine or sugar may be what you think you crave, but actually you need more! You need the power of God!

'A joyful heart makes a cheerful countenance,' reads the Proverbs. At the same time, a bad mood makes you tired.

Have you ever noticed how tiring it is to be angry or to think a lot of negative thoughts? That is because you were not created to think a lot of negative thoughts. You were created to meditate on the word of God and communicate with God himself.

As it is written in the book of Joshua, make your prayer: 'This book of the law shall not depart out of *my* mouth, but I shall meditate therein day and night, that *I* may observe to do according to all that is written therein; for then *I* will make my way prosperous, and then *I* shall have good success.'

One well-known preacher, previously a fat person, used to eat two or three large pies in one sitting. He was so fat he could hardly tie his shoes. He said he wouldn't have dreamed of stuffing himself with celery or cauliflower. That would be *punishment*.

What do reward and punishment mean to you? When you were a child, what were your favourite rewards? Were you rewarded with a 'treat' of sweets, biscuits, or ice cream? Do you do the same thing to your own children? When you give your child a treat, is it usually a sugar treat?

Punishment

What does punishment mean to you? Doesn't it mean being deprived of something? When you eat fattening foods you are depriving yourself of a beautiful body and a healthy mind.

The definition of punishment is: 'a penalty inflicted for an offence or fault'. You may think you are rewarding yourself by eating wrong foods, but you are really punishing yourself. You may joke about healthy low-calorie foods as punishment, but you have it confused. There's nothing at all punishing about proper eating.

The word of God gives you wisdom regarding the way you eat. The word of God makes you wise not foolish. You are no longer vain in your imaginings.

Your heart is not foolish, nor is it darkened. You're on the road to wisdom and beauty. You no longer profess yourself to be wise while actively showing yourself to be a fool (Rom 1:21b–22). You know the difference between punishment and reward.

In your diary, make a list of good things you'd like to have. Maybe it's a long, leisurely bubble bath, a long distance telephone call to a friend, curling up in your favourite chair and reading a good book (with the time gained through less eating). Maybe it's buying something or going somewhere. Maybe it's taking time off from a heavy schedule to do nothing at all, or work on a favourite hobby. On your list, do not mention foods.

Food is not a friend.

Be aware that the advertisements for food are for one purpose and one purpose only—to get your money. If you spend more time eating and preparing food than you do with Jesus, you have chosen the wrong friend. If you eat wherever you go and whenever you sit down, you've got the wrong companion. Jesus is your only true and faithful friend who loves you with the heart of eternity.

Food does not love you.

Love and food have nothing to do with one another. In spite of the fact that our celebrations and festive events are always accompanied by food and feasting, the food itself is not love. It is the *people* who represent the love. If you love food because it makes you feel loved just like when you were a small child when your mum used to feed you, it's your mum you ought to love and remember, not food! Your heart and mind ought to be fixed on loving and caring about *people*.

Food does not make you happy.

God is your happiness. Food is something to eat with care and dedication to the Lord in order to keep your body healthy, for he has given you your body to care for.

You use food, it doesn't use you.

You say to a cake, 'I don't want to put you into my body even though you'll taste good going down. You're no use to this body. I don't want you.' But you say to a big juicy apple, 'You would be useful to this body. You will also taste delicious. I want you.'

One lady returned from a church supper glowing with delight. Her friends were eager to learn how she had handled the affair.

'You should have seen all the food they spread out on the tables,' she said.

They nodded as people do while listening to unpleasant news.

'Everything was fattening. I mean, everything. As I passed along the length of the table I realized there was nothing I could eat. I was really hungry too. I would have loved to eat a few of those fattening fruit salad dishes with the whipped cream, telling myself, "Well, what else can I do? I have to eat *something*."'

If this hasn't happened to you yet, it will some time in the future. You will find yourself in circumstances that make it inconvenient to remain on your new eating habits. This woman handled it beautifully.

'I just said to all that food, "I don't want you. I won't eat you. You are fattening and have no nutritive value. I want to put food into this body that will make it run better."'

The others understood why she was glowing.

'So I had a pile of raw vegetables without dressing.'

You don't have to be a victim of circumstances. If

there's nothing but fattening food in front of you, change the circumstances. Nobody forces you to eat fattening food. If you eat it, you do so of your own choosing. You don't have to worry about insulting anybody. You don't have to worry about going hungry. You don't have to worry about being different.

Reward!

You can change your way of thinking about rewards. A reward should be something of *benefit* to you. Next time make sure dessert is something that's *good* for you!

Imagine you're sitting in a restaurant with somebody you really like and admire. Your friend looks at the menu and orders something greasy, fattening and with only a trace of vitamins or minerals, if any. You're stunned. (You always thought your friend was intelligent!) Then *you* look at the menu and order broiled fish with no butter and a large salad with fresh lemon juice as dressing. You've just given yourself a fabulous reward. A 'reward' is something given or received in return or recompense for service, merit, hardship, etc. You actually pay yourself for staying on your eating course and acting wisely.

You're out with slim friends who are eating disgustingly fattening foods, and you choose a green salad, and go without the rich dessert. By choosing the salad you thereby reward yourself. 'Wise choice,' you smile to yourself as you chew a piece of lettuce. 'I'm rewarded with good things and a slimmer body.'

You would have punished yourself by eating the rich dessert. You don't deserve to be punished. You deserve to be rewarded with good things, the good things that will make a happier and more beautiful you.

Listening to the Lord and obeying his voice is rewarding yourself. When you hear him tell you, 'Don't eat that,' and you obey, you can sing his praises and feel wonderful. When you hear him tell you, 'It's okay to eat that,' and you obey his directions, you receive a reward. Your reward is feeling good, blessed, happy, content, pleased. You are making Jesus Lord of your life. Jesus is now on the throne as ruler of your life, not you.

PRAYER

Dear Father, in the name of Jesus, I renounce the hold that food has had over me. I am now free by the power of the Holy Spirit within me.

Jesus died on the cross for me to set me free from the addiction to wrong foods. I refuse an attraction and interest in these foods in the name of Jesus.

Father, give me wisdom to understand the difference between reward and punishment. Help me to choose to reward my body, not punish it.

I do not blame my childhood or any person for my being overweight. I realize that nobody forces the fork into my mouth. I do it myself. Therefore I break the hold that past habits and experiences have had on me, tempting me to overeat and to eat sweets. Sweets are now ugly to me. I am free from them. They have made my body ugly and I refuse to give them that power over me any longer.

In Jesus' name, Amen.

Twelve

Knowing the Will of the Lord

My son [or my daughter], give attention to my words; incline your ear to my sayings. Do not let them depart from your sight; Keep them in the midst of your heart. For they are life to those who find them, and health to all their whole body (Prov 4:20–22).

Have you ever thought about the effect of obesity on your health? How many times have you visited someone with a highly contagious disease, such as hepatitis or even a streaming cold, and thrown your arms around them, hugging and kissing them? How many times have you asked to borrow the toothbrush of someone with the flu?

Those examples might sound unlikely, but millions of people every day harm their bodies in foolish ways. Think of the ways you have made your body fat and unhealthy. Consider the heaps of chips you've consumed in your lifetime, the pounds of chocolate, the rivers of ice cream. Our teeth, bones, liver, heart, skin and nerves show the damage.

The word of God leads us into health. The word of God *is* our health. If you love God, your love for your own body (the temple of the Holy Spirit) will motivate you to take good care of it.

> Put away from you a deceitful mouth, and put devious lips far from you (Prov 4:24).

The word of God does away with 'devious lips'; in our case, it's 'devious eating lips'.

The will of the Lord is that we live in honesty and truth. Our actions and deeds should not be hidden behind the larder door. The will of the Lord is that our lives be pure enough not to shame us at any time.

You can shout praises to the Lord, and sing, 'Hallelujah, Jesus is Lord of my life,' and then minutes later steal away to the refrigerator where you dip your finger in the trifle!

One woman shared how she sang, 'Take my life and let it be, consecrated Lord to thee...' in the morning church service, but that night lay on her bed sick from stuffing herself with food all day.

It is not God's will that we kill ourselves with a knife and fork. We were born to eat, not to diet or binge. It is God's will that our enemy, 'Lack of Discipline', be destroyed in us.

It is not God's will that we be addicted to junk food and sweets. Some people have their regular fix of biscuits, not unlike someone hooked on drugs. One of the differences is, the food junkie has a readier and cheaper supply at hand.

Eating the foods that Jesus would eat takes a little thought. Remember, we can be victims of advertising. Our source of nutritional knowledge shouldn't come from the magazines, TV and radio ads. If the wrapper on the bread says, 'Eat this; it's good for you,' don't buy it without reading what's in it. *You* decide if it's nutritious enough to eat.

Your will and God's!

'I've been dishonest with myself and God for years,' one woman shared. 'I know what it's like to not want to eat something and then eat it. I've even eaten things like the burnt biscuits out of the batch I'm baking just because I didn't want to throw them away. I mean, they taste awful. Yet I've eaten them.'

Devious lips devour burnt biscuits as if they didn't have calories. Devious lips also lick the finger after running it round the mixing bowl. Devious lips eat up the last of the food in the serving dishes while clearing the table. Devious lips gobble up the cake crumbs from around the cake.

Three or four burnt biscuits, a dollop of peanut butter and a handful of cake crumbs could add over 500 calories to your daily allowance. If you are on a 1,000 calorie a day diet, you have eaten half of your day's food and you may not have even counted it.

A deceitful mouth is a grumbling mouth. Deceit is lying. The devil 'is a liar, and the father of lies' (Jn 8:44). When you grumble, you are lying. You are saying things like, 'He is allowed to have a rich dessert and I have to eat cottage cheese. Who needs all this suffering? This is awful!'

The *truth* is, "Praise God, I'm eating beautiful cottage cheese and he's eating that sickly dessert. Thank God I do not have to eat the way he does. I can refrain. I can say no. Thank God for the power of the Holy Spirit dwelling in me. Thank you, Jesus, for strength and help.'

Remember your grateful heart will wash away the deceit of the enemy's lies. Your grateful heart won't allow your mouth to spew deceit. You won't lie, complain or grumble. Your grateful heart swells with love and gratitude, and even if you stumble, you can say,

'I'm sorry,' and pick yourself up again and start anew.

You say happily, 'Lord, I love you enough to eat 1,000 (or whatever) calories a day!' Don't plan any failures. You cannot lose with Jesus.

It is the will of the Lord that we are not defiled by the ways of the world. It is God's will that we...

> ...be filled with the knowledge of His will in all spiritual wisdom and understanding, so that you may walk in a manner worthy of the Lord, to please Him in all respects, bearing fruit in every good work and increasing in the knowledge of God; strengthened with all power, according to His glorious might, for the attaining of all steadfastness and patience; joyously (Col 1:9b–11).

Meditate on the above verses. They hold such magnificent promises and claims for us, we could spend a lifetime searching out their meaning and applying it to our lives.

Attaining 'steadfastness and patience joyously'— what words! They tell us that losing weight can be a joyous thing. We're attaining steadfastness by sticking to a calorie allowance and patience by seeing the pounds fall off far more slowly than we'd like them to. It's joyous!

When you are considering God's will for you, think about what his will is for *today*. Then, according to the above verse, as you are filled with the knowledge of his will in all spiritual wisdom and understanding, you know why obeying his will is important.

In your diary, on a separate page, draw a line down the centre of the paper. On one side, write, *God's will for me today is that I:* On the other side, write the spiritual wisdom and understanding you'll be gaining with the word *Why?*

Here is an example:

GOD'S WILL FOR ME TODAY	WHY?
1. Stay faithful to my calorie allowance.	To stay in close communication with him, so close that I lose the compulsion to overeat.
2. Fill in my calorie log daily.	
3. Be responsible for what I eat.	
4. Start today to take off the last 20lb to reach my goal weight.	To glorify him and be a beautiful witness of his power in my life.
5. Have a long quiet time with him and skip TV.	When I miss my daily quiet time or rush it, I don't soak in enough strength to overcome the temptation to overeat. (When I'm out of the word, I eat more.)
6. Do something creative that I enjoy (sewing, carpentry, pottery, painting, etc.).	To give me fun and relaxation, something I enjoy doing, and a sense of accomplishment. (I tend to eat when I feel bored or useless).
7. Finish a task that I've been putting off.	To remove frustration. (I eat when I'm frustrated, and unfinished work that piles up frustrates me.)

We know God's will by knowing his word. The more you meditate on the word, the more of him, his mind, his wisdom, his understanding, and his eternal purpose for your life you gain.

You can't obey his will unless you *know* his will. Jesus said, 'For whoever shall do the will of My Father who is in heaven, he is My brother and sister and mother' (Mt 12:50), showing us how close we can be to him *if* we know his will!

We learn his will from his word. In the word you learn how Jesus acted, spoke, prayed, thought. He is our model. He said, 'And He who sent Me is with Me; He has not left Me alone, for I always do the things that are pleasing to him' (Jn 8:29). It is his will that we be pleasing to him.

It is God's will that you gain wisdom and understanding in caring for your own body and the bodies of your loved ones.

Good food

The foods that have defiled our bodies are foods that have appealed to our flesh, not our spirit. The Bible tells us that we are living in a world dominated by sin, but we are born-again creatures, 'not of this world', and not to be *dominated* by the world and its ways.

Jesus prayed to his Father in John 17, 'I have given them [you and me] Thy word; and the world has hated them, because they are not of the world, even as I am not of the world' (v 14).

Do you think that bag of Liquorice Allsorts in the sweet shop has your name on it? Are the smells coming from that fish and chip shop calling you *personally* to their doors?

Jesus prayed to the Father not to remove those beckoning smells and sights from you, but to *keep you from succumbing*.

> I do not ask Thee to take them out of the world, but to keep them from the evil one. They are not of the world, even as I am not of the world (Jn 17:15–16).

Alice used to bake biscuits for the family and then eat them all herself before the children arrived home from school. When the children walked in the door, they could smell biscuits, but couldn't find them. Alice had to quickly whip up some more in order not to face the disgrace of what she had done.

God so loved the *world* (you and me who live in the world and are living in the midst of its ways and influences) that he sent his only Son, Jesus, to die on the cross for us and by believing in him, have eternal life and power and strength to live each day above the cares of this world.

The world offers a lot of rubbish to put into your body. It even offers supposedly low-calorie products that are just as harmful to your body as sugars, starches and processed foods. Artificial sweeteners, chemicals, additives, preservatives, etc., have long been the outrage of nutritionists who publish lengthy tomes on their dangers to the human body.

If you're accustomed to putting sugar in your hot drink, please don't switch to saccharin or a chemical sugar substitute. Try to eat more natural sugar from fresh fruit. Try cooking with honey, for example, (count the calories, though! One tablespoon of honey equals 65 calories), or fresh fruit juices.

Be of good cheer. Jesus has overcome the world. He has overcome sugar, sweets, starches, chemical sweeteners—the substances that load your veins with cholesterol and crowd your organs with fat and disease.

> For all that is in the world, the lust of the flesh and the lust of the eyes and the boastful pride of life, is not from the Father, but is from the world. And the world is passing away, and also its lusts; but the one who does the will of God abides forever (1 Jn 2:16–17).

Maybe at one time you loved junk food and sweets and you were fat because of them, but now you are free to love healthy food and be slim because of it.

> Do not love the world, nor the things in the world. If any one loves the world, the love of the Father is not in him (1 Jn 2:15).

You are a child of God. You are now free to eat foods that feed your body and make it strong. The whole world lies in the power of the evil one, but you are no longer a victim of the world and its fattening foods.

Protein foods:

Fish (without batter or breadcrumbs), fresh or frozen, broiled or baked, or steamed
Tinned tuna, salmon, sardines
Chicken (without the skin) or turkey, broiled, baked or steamed
Fresh eggs poached, boiled, scrambled with cheese
Cottage cheese (low calorie)
Cheeses
Lean meats
Wholemeal breads, rolls and cereals
Wheat germ, bran

Vitamin and mineral feasts:

Fresh vegetables of all kinds served in dozens of fabulous salad combinations
Homemade dressings prepared with natural ingredients
Cooked or steamed vegetables, eaten hot and crisp without butter (or very little)
Beautiful fresh fruit of every kind eaten raw or cooked in a variety of delightful combinations or eaten singly
Drinks of fresh fruit or vegetable juices without added sugar.

We are no longer ignorant of the harmful effects of sugar and artificial sweeteners on our bodies. This information isn't a secret any more. It's a known fact that overdoses of artificial sweeteners cause cancer in laboratory animals. Extended use in the diets of children could lead to cancer in their adult years. Before you throw your hands in the air and yell, 'There's nothing we can eat any more! Everything causes cancer!' let's take the matter to the Lord. What do these facts mean to us as Christians and what does the Lord say to us about them?

We're telling you to stop eating harmful foods, but we ask you to talk to the Lord about your responsibility in the light of the known facts.

You ought to feel good about yourself. The Lord loves you so wonderfully. 'My love and kindness shall not depart from you, nor shall My covenant of peace and completeness be removed, says the Lord, Who has compassion on you' (Is 54:10 AMP).

Feel good about yourself and don't take the fun out of eating. Enjoy healthy vitamin-rich foods. Let your body, soul and spirit glorify the Lord.

PRAYER

Thank you, Jesus, for food that makes my body alive with vitality and strength. Thank you, Jesus, for food that builds muscles, restores worn tissues, make bones, teeth, gums, hair and skin healthy and strong.

Thank you, Jesus, for power to overcome the attraction to the world's foods.

Thank you, Jesus, for the power of your word in my life. Thank you for your promises now coming true in my life. Thank you for your wonderful word which has become health to my whole body, just as you said it would.

Amen.

Thirteen

Budgeting Calories and Nutrition

Now that you're able to resist wrong foods, you'll want to budget your calories in food groups. Decide how many calories you're going to spend on protein for the day, how many on fruit, vegetables, juices.

It's necessary to know the nutritive content of foods to know the best sources of various nutrients that your body needs. The more varied your diet the better. *All* nutrients are essential for good health and nutrition.

A common error dieters make in meal planning is emphasizing one type of food and excluding others. If you concentrate your diet on only one or two types of foods, you'll suffer a lack of necessary elements, including protein, fats, carbohydrates, mineral salts and vitamins, all vitally necessary for your body to function smoothly.

As tissues are broken down in your body, the wastes are eliminated and the tissues replaced and replenished by the foods you eat. If one essential element is missing from your diet, your health will suffer.

Protein (fish, eggs, chicken, turkey, cheese, cottage cheese, lean meats) supplies muscle-forming elements and acts as fuel for energy. Carbohydrates and fats (protein foods, whole grain foods, natural sugars) provide heat and energy to the body system and influence protein metabolism. Vitamins and minerals (fruits and vegetables) are crucial in keeping the metabolism in good working order.

Protein

The word protein is derived from a Greek word meaning 'to take first place'. Protein foods are of first importance in the diet. Your body needs the carbohydrate and fat found in protein-rich foods. (This doesn't mean the grease from sausages or beefburgers or the melted butter on your jacket potato. There is absolutely no protein in butter or grease.)

Some proteins are superior in quality to others. For example, fish, which is close to meat in protein content, has been found to be superior in protein quality.

The best sources of protein are animal sources such as milk, eggs, cheese, meat, poultry and fish for highest biological value. Three of these foods alone can provide 51g of protein. They are a pint of milk, an egg and 100g of meat or meat substitutes (fish, poultry, cheese). Grains such as wheat, soy beans, corn, rice, as well as nuts, peas, beans, lentils and peanuts provide a second source of protein.

Weight-loss diets that advocate eating only protein foods are not wise to follow. They not only rob your body of the valuable vitamins and minerals it needs to function properly, but nutritionists consider excess protein a health hazard due to the uric acid and toxic substances that produce fermentation in the body. Too much protein results in putrification in the body. Too much carbohydrate produces fermentation. (You can see why God admonishes us to avoid excesses!)

Nutritional awareness

It is important that you have nutritional awareness. Misinformation abounds left and right. Suppose one day someone tells you banana skins are a miracle food and eating thirty a day will add years to your life. The next day you may hear that if you eat watermelon seeds every day, your hair will grow thicker and longer. Or suppose someone tells you sugar won't hurt you; it just flushes right through the body. Or you hear, 'You don't need protein three times a day,' or 'It's okay to skip meals. You lose weight that way,' or 'Taking vitamin supplements won't help the body at all.' All of theses are not only humorous, but incorrect.

It's important that you know what's going on nutritionally so that you develop your own diet in wisdom and truth. In order for your body to be healthy and strong, you need to be informed and intelligent about food and its nutrients. Health and your for ever-thin body won't happen by accident. You make it happen.

A common malady of fat people is that they do not *want* to know about nutrition because it may mean they'll have to change their buying and eating habits. You are now past that point in your new road to slimness and health. You have already committed yourself to losing weight. Now you are learning how to do it wisely. You are learning how to bless your own body.

You are becoming aware of: How the body functions utilize each food nutrient, and what the body requirements are for optimum health and vitality.

Below is a daily food guide published by the U.S. Department of Agriculture. It shows you clearly that each nutrient is important to your health.

A DAILY FOOD GUIDE

Milk Group (8-ounce cups)

2 to 3 cups for children under nine years
3 or more cups for children nine to twelve years
4 cups or more for teenagers
2 cups or more for adults
3 cups or more for pregnant women
4 cups or more for nursing mothers

Meat Group

Two or more servings. Count as one serving:

2 or 3 ounces lean, cooked beef, veal, pork, lamb, poultry, fish—without bone
2 eggs
1 cup cooked dry beans, dry peas, lentils
4 tablespoons peanut butter

Vegetable/Fruit Group
(1/2 cup serving or 1 piece of fruit, etc.)

Four or more servings per day, including:

1 serving of citrus fruit, or other fruit or vegetable as a good source of vitamin C, or 2 servings of a fair source
1 serving, at least every other day, of a dark-green or deep-yellow vegetable for vitamin A
2 or more servings of other vegetables and fruits, including potatoes

Breads/Cereals Group

Four or more servings daily (whole-grain, enriched or restored). Count as one serving:

1 slice bread
1 ounce ready-to-eat cereal

½ to ¾ cup cooked cereal, cornmeal, macaroni, noodles, rice or spaghetti.

'Consumers All Yearbook of Agriculture, 1965,' U.S. Department of Agriculture, Washington, D.C., 1965, p.394.

Overeaters Victorious recommends a diet guideline adaptable to any daily calorie limit. You will find it an introduction to a simple way to eat. It is found at the end of this book. You may want to use this to guide your daily calorie allowance. It is important to eat a balanced diet each day. It is important you don't skip meals. Each meal you eat (particularly a high-protein meal) increases metabolism and burns up fat deposits. By eating three high-protein, low-fat meals, you actually lose weight faster than if you skipped meals or went on a starvation diet. Protein three times a day keeps your blood sugar level high and aids in preventing hunger pangs. Your body makes use of the food you eat in a steady, timed manner when you eat three meals a day. Worn out tissues are repaired, energy is released and utilized and your body functions in an orderly way, as God planned it to.

PRAYER

Dear Lord, help me to develop an interest in nutrition and what my body needs to function smoothly for your glory. I choose to be wise in my eating habits and I choose your wisdom in the foods I put into my body.

I confess and renounce my old habits of eating too much of one food to the exclusion of another. I confess and renounce skipping meals and then binging at the next one. I was ignorant about nutrition and how to eat. I was lazy and irresponsible in food preparation. I bought foods through lust and greed rather than in wisdom and understanding, and I renounce the lusts for those foods that are harmful to my body.

I refuse to be a friend of the world's system and foods. I choose to eat good food to the glory of God. In Jesus' name, Amen!

Submit therefore to God. Resist the devil and he will flee from you (Jas 4:7).

Fourteen

How to Exercise Self-control When You Don't Think You Have Any

Carolyn was once a heavy smoker and smoked as many as five packets of cigarettes a day. She also drank heavily. When she became a Christian she gave her life to the Lord, allowing him to work his will in her. She wanted to be free from smoking and drinking. She mentioned how the Lord marvellously helped her overcome her smoking habit. She prayed and asked him to deliver her from the cigarettes and he did. She went from five packets a day to none.

The next thing she wanted to be rid of in her life was the drinking. She knew that if she didn't stop, she could well become an alcoholic. Drinking had become a lifestyle and she enjoyed it too much to be safely within the limits of moderation.

So she simply stopped. She drinks fruit and vegetable juices now. 'I can't say it was really that hard to stop smoking and drinking,' she said. 'I gave these things up for Jesus and I felt really good about it.'

But Carolyn is morose and depressed, and telling herself she is a failure. 'I have no self-control. I'm overweight and I just can't seem to stop eating.'

You can see how wrong she is. With the Lord's help she has successfully got rid of two enormous strongholds in her life. Now she has an opportunity to get rid of a third. But instead of seeing her weight problem as an opportunity, she saw it as a curse.

Helen had a habit of using foul language. She swore and cursed with such a rapid flow of filth that even she would be repulsed. 'It was awful. I cursed every time I opened my mouth. I gave my heart to Jesus and at first nothing changed. Then gradually, as I asked him to help me stop swearing, he began to help me. I worked at it and totally stopped. Thank God, I'm free. It was like living in hell and speaking its language.'

But Helen despairs over her 1½st of extra weight. 'I just don't seem to have any self-control,' she says.

We need to understand three things about self-control. Firstly, God is the giver of all gifts and the fruit of the Spirit is accomplished by his presence within you. Fruit is accomplished, not given. Self-control is a fruit of the Holy Spirit.

Secondly, when we ask God to do something in our lives, he will do it with our consent and effort. (See chapter 12.) If you ask God to get you to church on time, he can't very well do it if you don't get out of bed when he awakens you.

Self-control is saying to yourself, 'Get out of bed.'

Thirdly, self-control is something you exercise every day of your life. *You* are in control of your *self*. In order to read this book, you had to pick it up, you had to turn the pages, you had to put your eyes on the pages and decipher the words. You exercised *control* of your *self* and did these things. Nobody else did them for you. If someone is reading this book to you, it's your ears doing the listening. You are in control.

If you think you have no self-control in your life because you're overweight, take a look at some other areas in your life where you do exercise self-control. For example, do you get out of bed when the alarm clock rings, arrive at work on time, and brush your teeth?

If the answer is yes, then you can see how you do *not* lack self-control in your life at all.

List some of the bad habits and fleshly indulgences that you have already given up in your life (i.e. drugs, smoking, drinking, swearing, lying, gossiping, cheating, stealing, biting your nails, bed-wetting, thumb-sucking, scratching, oversleeping, habitual lateness, lustful thoughts, etc.) Take time to think about this list. If you can put *one* thing on your list, you have proved that you *do* have self-control.

Now let's make this self-control work for you in the area of your weight.

Overeating belongs in the same camp of indulgences as those on the previous list. When Carolyn says, 'I have victory in the areas of smoking and drinking, but not in eating,' she is not quite accurate. The truth is, she has victory in all three because they are, in fact, one area. If you can stop smoking and drinking you can stop overeating. Some people, however, continue to overeat because they are really *still* smoking and drinking *through* the overeating.

You *do* have self-control. You're lying to yourself if you say you don't. When you read verses in the Bible that say, 'Watch over your heart with all diligence, for from it flow the springs of life,' and, 'Let your eyes look directly ahead, and let your gaze be fixed straight in front of you' (Prov 4:23,25), you are reading about self-control. When you make a decision, any decision, you are exercising self-control. When you exert effort to do something that is difficult to do, you are exercising self-control.

What gives me self-control?

Please realize that you do have self-control. You use your self-control every day in some way or other. God brings self-control into your life through a variety of ways. Some of these ways you might not like, but some of them you will. Thank God for the privilege to learn self-control!

Psalm 119:65–68 says:

> Thou hast dealt well with Thy servant, O Lord, according to Thy word.

In his word is everything we could possibly need in this life to teach us and guide us into every fulfilment and joy. He does deal well with us.

> Teach me good discernment and knowledge, for I believe in Thy commandments.

Teach me, Lord, why it is I could stop biting my fingernails, but I can't stop overeating.

> Before I was afflicted I went astray.

Before I piled all this fat on my body, I went far away from self-control and godliness and overate.

> But now I keep Thy word.

Your word to me is that you want me to eat___calories a day and lose___pounds.

> Thou art good and doest good.

Thank you, Jesus, that you forgive me when I fail.

Teach me Thy statutes.

I'm desperate enough and afflicted with enough fat now to want to hear your voice and your will for my body.

It is good for me that I was afflicted, that I may learn Thy statutes (Ps 119:71).

I never dreamed there'd be anything good about being fat, but Lord, it has brought me to this point in my life with you where I am willing to learn your will, your law, your rules. It is good for me that I gained weight so that through being overweight and fat, I can become a far more powerful Christian than I otherwise would have chosen to be.

One woman paraphrased verse 71 to read, 'Because I am fat, I am now learning about self-control. I can arrive at the maturity held out to me from the Lord *faster* than if I were not fat. It is good for me that I have been afflicted with fat in order that I can reach such a wonderful close position with God.'

This is a beautiful place to be with the Lord. 'I shall delight in Thy statutes' (Ps 119:16a) is your new life-song. You delight with your glass of water when everyone else is eating chocolate cake. You delight in your lean meat, broiled chicken, fish, fresh vegetables and fruits, fresh eggs and cheeses. What a *delight* to weigh in each week and see God chiselling the fat off your body.

The way to exercise self-control when you don't think you have any is:

Realize you do have self-control.

It's simply untrue that you have no self-control. You

exercise self-control every day of your life. You are exercising self-control right now by reading this book. You're telling yourself what to do and you are doing it.

Stop being hard on yourself.

God knows your frame. He knows that you are a human being and endowed with human characteristics. 'He regards the lowly,' it says in Psalm 138:6. 'He remembered us in our low estate' (Ps 136:23). 'The Lord preserves the simple: I was brought low, and He saved me' (Ps 116:6).

David agonized in plea after plea for the Lord to rescue him from his troubles and weaknesses. He knew that he couldn't win any battle or overcome any struggle without the help of the Lord. He knew it because he knew that as a human being, he simply wasn't equipped to do it in his own strength.

The Lord tells us this dramatic truth, that [his] strength is made perfect in weakness (2 Cor. 12:9 AV).

'Let the weak say I am strong!' he shouts from heaven (Joel 3:10 AV).

Rejoice in the self-control you do have.

Pat yourself on the back every time you move the plate of biscuits away from you. Every time you order a salad when everyone else is eating something rich and calorie-laden, celebrate your wise choice by a long and leisurely good thought about yourself. Every time you push yourself away from the table instead of eating dessert, rejoice.

When is the last time you said, 'I did it!' or 'Good for me!' ? Start saying these things about yourself.

You *do* have self-control!

PRAYER

Thank you, dear Jesus, for the self-control that I *do* have. Thank you, dear Jesus, that the self-control in my life is accomplished by your presence within me.

Now, in the name of Jesus, I choose to exercise this fruit of the Holy Spirit in a more dynamic way than ever before in my life. I unleash God-given strengths and abilities so far unused within me and call upon self-control to show itself prominently in my life.

I choose to exercise self-control in the area of food!

In Jesus' name, I am victorious over temptation! Amen.

Fifteen

What to Do When You Blow It

What happened? You say you prayed for self-control and made a list of food you wouldn't ever allow to touch your lips again, and then you—you—oh, no, you ate *what*?

You're feeling miserable, your face is covered with guilt. Your stomach is sick, your head is sick, your toes are sick. You would just like to curl up into a ball and turn into a doorknob.

What's the use? you wonder. All is hopeless. All is defeat and doom. 'Oh, God, why was I born?' you ask. If you haven't said it, you're thinking it. What a horrible cross to bear—this overeating problem. Why doesn't God just remove it from me? Where is he when I need him?

What misery and rottenness!

Now, wait a minute. So you blew it, and it's not the first time, you say. You failed last week, too, and the week before that.

Well, that certainly proves one thing, doesn't it? You are a human being and human beings are, in themselves, weak. It also proves that you have the strength to pick yourself up and start all over again because the Lord tells us, 'Let the weak say I am strong.'

You can't do that, you say? Feeling too rotten. In fact, you feel so rotten, you'd like to eat something. That way the guilt you are already feeling would have some more guilt to keep it company. Then you could be even more miserable than you are right now. The more miserable you feel, the more you eat. The more you eat, the more miserable you feel.

Imagine walking past one of your previously favourite bakers. In days gone by you couldn't resist going in, buying something and eating it. But now since you've begun your new diet, you haven't gone into that bakers once and you haven't eaten anything of theirs. You've had wonderful self-control. But today it's past lunch-time and you didn't have much breakfast and bakery smells are thick in the air....

A tempting voice at your ear says to you, 'Why not have something from the bakers? It won't hurt you. Go on. You can count it as your lunch. Besides, you had such a small breakfast. Don't you feel weak? Of course you do. What you need is a little sustenance inside you.'

You try to protest. 'But I made a commitment. I—I—.' Now you're passing the door. The little voice at your ear says, 'Look at those fresh things in the window. No, don't turn your head. What harm can a little peep do? Look! Your favourite! Remember in the old days how you could eat dozens of those at a time?'

You turn, you look, you crave. You're salivating now. 'That's right,' says the little voice; 'don't they look *delicious*? Why not go inside? You could buy something to take home for the family!'

That did it. Of course! You'll do it for the others! So you dash into the shop, your eyes ablaze with excitement. You buy an armful of goodies and stumble out, telling yourself how nice you are to think of others before yourself.

By the next corner you've already eaten two

chocolate-covered doughnuts, and by the time you get to the bus stop or to your car, you've polished off half the iced buns too.

The little voice at your ear isn't saying much now, but once in a while between chomps you think you hear unpleasant laughter.

By the time you get home, you've eaten the cake and the sausage rolls. There are only two doughnuts left. How can you go in with only two doughnuts—plain at that. You wouldn't want to do that. There's no alternative but to eat them too. So before getting out of the car, you wolf down the last two doughnuts.

Now the voice at your ear returns. There it is, loud and clear. You hear it as you stagger like a drunk into your house. *'Now* you've done it, fatso!' You listen miserably. 'Oh, now I've done it,' you repeat.

The voice sneers, 'You haven't got a shred of self-control in you! You're a total failure! You blew it! What a tub of lard you are! Oh, you'll pay for this binge, all right!'

You are utterly crushed and condemned.

You don't want to talk to anyone or even see anyone. You're nauseous and dizzy. You hurt all over. You just want to crash into bed and sleep for ever. Or sit down and stare at the TV.

Do you see the pattern in all this? The devil, who is the father of lies, roars around like a lion seeking whom he can devour with those lies of his. He appeals to your flesh, the weak part of you. Then, when you fall prey to his lies, he shrieks with torrents of condemning words. He'll call you names; he'll say how disgusting you are; how unloved, how hopeless, how fat and ugly. He'll tell you nobody loves you, you're miserable and will always be miserable. He's got you where he wants you—right in the position where you'll listen to him and believe every word he tells you.

If Satan can cause you to feel wretchedly guilty, he's got you in his clutches. For this reason it's very important that you recognize his tactics. All right, you blew it. So what? Pick yourself up and carry on. Your diet is not geared to last for just a couple of weeks or months. It is a lifelong commitment. No matter how many times you blow it, you're not going to give up. So you blew it at breakfast. Go back on the diet at lunch. Write down in your journal the calories you eat, no matter how many.

Remember, overeating can be one of the traits of rebellion and selfishness. You may not *want* to write down the calories amount on your binge. Maybe you rebel at the idea. It's okay, the Lord is with you and he loves you in spite of everything. With this knowledge, the devil will not be able to continue his disgusting game. He'll see that you're not going to sink into guilt and despair every time you blow it. You're confessing your sins to God and you're refusing to hate yourself. God wants you to love yourself. The devil wants you to hate yourself.

God tells us to love our neighbours as *ourselves;* that means we should have an abundance of healthy, sound love for ourselves first. As a result of this love, we love others. God wants you to love yourself, and because you belong to him, you naturally want what he wants. You belong to God. You are his. You're not something for the devil to manipulate like a plaything.

The Lord is saying to you:

Do not fear, for I am with you;
Do not anxiously look about you, for I am your God.
I will strengthen you, surely I will help you.
Surely I will uphold you with My righteous right hand
(Is 41:10).

He is right there with you. As you confess what you did, asking for his forgiveness, he is right there to forgive you!

He forgives all your sins for the asking. Every calorie that you eat beyond your allowance, every crumb you sneak into your mouth, every time you cheat, every lie that you have told yourself and believed, every indulgence, *everything*.

He forgives.

If we confess our sins, He is faithful and righteous to forgive us our sins and to cleanse us from all unrighteousness (1 Jn 1:9).

I, even I, am he that blotteth out thy transgressions for mine own sake, and will not remember thy sins (Is 43:25 AV).

I have wiped out your transgressions like a thick cloud, and your sins like a heavy mist. Return to Me, for I have redeemed you (Is 44:22).

Return unto him. It's okay, return and go on with the diet. If you overate at 10:30 in the morning, don't tell yourself you'll go back on your diet tomorrow; do it at lunch! Count your calories and have a good lunch within your calorie limit. Don't skip meals and try to atone for your sins.

Trying to atone for overindulgence

Binging followed by fasting is a familiar syndrome. Binge/Fast. Binge/Fast. Before long it becomes Binge/Binge.

You think it's all right to snack on something fattening between meals because you just won't eat dinner.

Not true.

It is not okay to snack on something fattening between meals and it is not all right to go without dinner. You cannot atone for your own sins.

Jesus Christ is our atonement for sins. You can't atone for them yourself. You are learning how to *eat*, not fast. It may take some struggles and a few ups and downs, but it's all in the process of getting that flesh of yours under control. You've been a rebellious person, selfish and uncommitted to the Lord in your eating habits. You're making progress, but sometimes the going gets a little choppy.

You want to lose weight faster than it wants to get lost. Those great claims made by promoters of fad diets or weight-loss clinics, telling you that in 30 days you'll be 2st lighter; or by Christmas, your birthday, Aunt Maude's housewarming or your own wedding day, you'll be a sliver of your former fat ugly self, are not only unsound, but unhealthy. We said earlier don't fast to lose weight when you are in the process of learning how to *eat*. It may throw your whole metabolism out of order and later you'll weigh more than you do at the moment.

Obese people often choose radical weight-loss methods that harm their bodies and destroy their health because of a mistaken notion that doing something radical will somehow atone for the sins that caused them to be fat. Selfishness makes patience hard to come by.

You want to be 2st slimmer and you want it *now*. The sooner the better, so naturally, when some promoter comes along telling you that you can lose so much weight in a short time, you're going to reach into your pocket and pay whatever they ask to have this dream come true in your life.

The sad thing is, the dream doesn't come true. You may lose weight, but statistics have shown, if you don't

learn new *eating* habits, the weight doesn't stay off.
Don't be like the young woman who drank predigested
liquid protein and lost 4½st, but damaged her heart
and metabolism so that she will never be normal again.

Don't try to atone for your own sins. Jesus is your
atonement. He went to the cross, carrying your fat with
him, so that you could overcome overeating and be
victorious!

Long-suffering

Long-suffering is another fruit of the Spirit. When you
think of long-suffering, you think of patience. *Be patient
with yourself*. It will take longer to get back on your
weight-loss course if you condemn yourself. If you
have patience and compassion, you will be able to pick
yourself up and start again without wasting too much
time in self-pity and condemnation.

> There is therefore now no condemnation for those who are
> in Christ Jesus (Rom 8:1).

Remember that.

Long-suffering towards yourself means demonstrat-
ing mercy and compassion. You don't go to pieces
when you blow it; you ask forgiveness and start again.
Long-suffering exhibits tolerance, humanity, charity,
and tenderness—towards yourself as well as towards
others.

Probably one of the reasons you overeat is that you
dislike yourself. You need to fight this by being kind to
yourself. Whatever you do, reject condemnation.

Jim tells how he was once hooked on Pepsi Cola. He
drank a minimum of a dozen cans a day. Most of the
time he drank more than that. He prayed and prayed
for help. He asked friends to pray for him, too, but

nothing seemed to work. He just couldn't break his habit. His stomach, teeth, and skin were suffering terribly—he had chronic acne, his teeth were fast decaying and his stomach burned so badly he thought he was getting an ulcer.

Then one day he said, 'That's it. This is the last Pepsi I'm drinking,' and he gave it up. Within a week, he was feeling better and knew he was rid of the habit for ever.

A short time later he began to pray about losing weight. He was 3½st overweight. He began the OV course and lost 9lb the first week. The weight loss was slower after that and one week he gained 5lb. He despaired and sank into a mood of defeat.

'But you conquered the Pepsi habit!' the members of his group reminded him. 'You're a success! You're not a failure! Why are you despairing?'

It is so easy to forget our triumphs and concentrate on our failures. Long-suffering gives us patience with ourselves.

Jim did not fast to lose the added 5lb and he did not go without lunches for a week, as he wanted to. The weight came off slower than he would have liked, but it came off eventually and permanently.

> All discipline for the moment seems not to be joyful, but sorrowful; yet to those who have been trained by it, after-wards it yields the peaceful fruit of righteousness. There-fore, strengthen the hands that are weak and the knees that are feeble, and make straight paths for your feet, so that the limb which is lame may not be put out of joint, but rather be healed (Heb 12:11–13).

Maybe this is the first time in your life you've had an opportunity to learn how to be patient with yourself, kind to yourself, gentle to yourself, long-suffering towards yourself.

You need long-suffering to be a successful Christian.

You need it so that if you make a mistake, you don't hate yourself, but you have mercy on yourself.

PRAYER

I am a born-again child of God. Thank you, Father for your great love and mercy. Thank you for sending Jesus to die on the cross so that I don't have to atone for my own sins.

Thank you for your Holy Spirit enabling me to have mastery over my flesh. I refuse to be a selfish person! I have self-control!

Thank you for developing long-suffering and patience in me. Thank you, Lord, for freeing me from self-condemnation. I can be patient, kind and understanding towards myself!

Thank you, Lord, that you do not expect me to conquer all my faults in one day. I am not discouraged at my progress because you are my judge and enabler!

In Jesus' name and for him. Amen.

Sixteen

Look Where You Are!

Becky had had a great week. She didn't go over her calorie allowance once. She wrote down everything she ate and its calorie content on her log sheet in her notebook. She was so pleased with herself she even started doing physical exercises.

Then she received a jolt of disappointment when she weighed in. Her weight loss for the week was only 4oz.

Talk about discouraging.

Her friend, Linda, had one of the best weeks since beginning her course. She hadn't missed one day's quiet time with Jesus, she recorded her calories faithfully, and she stayed within her calorie allowance throughout the entire week.

When she weighed in she had *gained* ½lb.

Where is justice? you wonder. Both Becky and Linda had worked hard, remained faithful (God knows it wasn't easy to say no to little Billy's hardly-touched plate of chips). Is there no reward for such faithful sacrifice?

These girls had a choice, just as you do at times like this when you work hard and don't lose the weight you expected to.

Becky and Linda can either feel angry, hurt and

defeated (all of which cause overeating) or they can praise the Lord for the victory they won throughout the week by being faithful (which brings you closer to Jesus and gives you a good feeling about yourself).

When you feel good about yourself and the world around you, you don't overeat.

Becky and Linda did choose to rejoice. They praised the Lord for the power to remain faithful in spite of temptations and in spite of not losing as much as they hoped to that week. They also praised the Lord that other people had big weight losses that week, and that way they avoided jealously and frustration.

'I'm victorious!' is the truth they repeatedly said. They knew words like 'What's the use? I'm doomed to be fat' were lies.

Perhaps you tell yourself some of the following lies?

- What's the use? I'm doomed to be fat.
- I'll never lose weight, no matter how hard I try.
- I pray, but God doesn't help me.
- God must be punishing me for my sins. They're too terrible for him to forgive.
- I lose weight, but then I regain it straight away. I'll never be permanently slim.
- God must be sick of my losing weight, regaining it, and then losing it again. He has definitely lost his patience with me.

All of these statements are lies. You are *not* doomed to be fat. You *will* lose weight. God *does* help you. Nothing is too terrible for God to forgive! You *will* lose weight and keep it off. God will never lose patience with you. *Trust* him.

No matter how many times you exceed your calorie allowance or go off your course God will never give up on you! Start again!

Jean is a woman who started her course in the spring, fell away during the summer, started again in the autumn, blew it at Christmas, started again in January, fell away in April, started again in September; at the moment she's still going strong. She's lost a total of 2½st since she began. If she had stuck to the course continuously she'd be at her goal weight by now, but she is rejoicing at what the Lord is teaching her and doing in her life through her times of stumbling.

You don't overcome that rebellious nature and those rebellious habits overnight.

If you stumble, get up and carry on! Continue with *Jesus*. Get your nose back into the Bible. Eat your spiritual life-giving food!

In 2 Chronicles 16, it tells how King Asa of Judah went to the King of Syria with gifts of gold and silver, pleading for his help against the King of Israel. The King of Syria obliged and conquered some of Israel's store cities in Naphtali. Then the King of Judah wiped out the work Israel was doing in building Ramah.

It looked like King Asa had really had everything going on his side. He had big armies and he had destroyed the enemy's stronghold. But in the middle of all his victory, God sent a prophet to him who told him. 'You've made a mistake, Asa. God never intended for you to rely on some other king!'

'You mean the King of Syria to whom I turned for help?'

'That's right. God is saying, "Because you have relied on the King of Syria and have not relied on the Lord your God, you didn't conquer what you were supposed to conquer at all."'

King Asa didn't like what he was hearing. He had a rebellious heart. He wanted to do things *his* way.

'Asa, listen to me,' the prophet continued. 'The eyes of the Lord move to and fro throughout the earth that he may strongly support those whose heart is completely his. You have acted foolishly in this.'

Why do we turn to fad diets, fasts, pills, drugs, shots, powdered drinks, and occult practices to lose weight? These all fail before they begin. *God does not fail.*

Asa sounds like a familiar character. (We may wonder if he had a weight problem!) He wanted to depend on himself and his own ways and not on God.

What usually happens when you trust yourself and not God? If you fail, you get angry. That's what Asa did. He was furious. He threw the prophet in jail and took his wrath out on some of the people.

He didn't want to win his battles God's way. He didn't want God's power and God's overcoming strength. He wanted *his* way. (Our way is to eat whatever and whenever we want with nobody to get in our way.)

King Asa could have repented and started again. But he didn't. He refused to repent. (That's what a long food binge is like. After the first ten minutes, each additional mouthful of food is a refusal to repent.) Asa absolutely refused to repent and start again with the Lord.

So he failed—and failed miserably at that. He became diseased in his feet and in verse 12 it says his disease was really severe. But even *then* he wouldn't turn to the Lord for help. Do you know whom he turned to? Some physicians. That's like some obese people who are so sick with obesity that they overeat even more. (See chapter 17.)

No matter how slow the weight loss is, don't give up. Even if you gain weight, don't give up. Many people will lose weight and then regain some, but if you stick with it, you'll lose more than you gained and you'll be nearer your goal.

You are at a very important place in your life. See

Ephesians 1:3–14 and look where you are.

> Blessed be the God and Father of our Lord Jesus Christ, who has blessed us with every spiritual blessing in the heavenly places in Christ.

You are not only blessed once or twice, but with *every* spiritual blessing in heavenly places in Christ. When you're with Christ, you are in heavenly places, whether standing at the door of the refrigerator or on your knees in prayer. Your heart and your mind belong to him to bless with *every* spiritual blessing. His spiritual blessings are eternal. They are heavenly. You are not hopeless, or a failure in Christ. You are *blessed*.

> Just as He chose us in Him before the foundation of the world that we should be holy and blameless before Him.

You are chosen! You're not somebody sitting on the fringe of the heavenly crowd wishing you could be a part of it. You *are* in there! You're *chosen*!

> In love He predestined us to adoption as sons [daughters too] through Jesus Christ to Himself, according to the kind intention of His will.

You are adopted by him. He has picked you to father, to take care of, to raise and love. His intentions towards you are loving and kind.

> To the praise of the glory of His grace, which He freely bestowed on us in the Beloved.

His grace and his unfailing and unmerited mercy are lavished upon you.

> In Him we have redemption through His blood, the for-

giveness of our trespasses, according to the riches of His grace.

Do you know what it is to be really forgiven? Forgiven for every second and third helping your body didn't need, every gorging and binging experience? Do you know what it is to be forgiven for the causes of your overeating?

Have you ever asked the Lord to *forgive* you for those feelings of frustration, or for the mistaken notion that life is passing you by, and you're missing out on happiness and beauty?

Riches in grace mean rich in forgiveness, renewing, healing, restoring, blessing. Redemption means to be bought back from the rightful owner. We have redemption through the blood he bled when he was hung on the cross and we're forgiven!

Which He lavished upon us. In all wisdom and insight.

You're not foolish. You have wisdom and insight! Use it!

He made known to us the mystery of His will, according to His kind intention which He purposed in Him.

(If you think you just can't figure out what God's will is for you, read this verse again.) He has made the mystery of his will known to us! It says so right here. Believe it. Pray, 'Lord, I take the power to know the mystery of your will just as it says in this ninth verse of Ephesians 1.'

Also we have obtained an inheritance, having been predestined according to His purpose who works all things after the counsel of His will.

That's good news. Do you know what it is to receive an inheritance? That means somebody *gives* you something; you inherit it. If you had a distant uncle who left you a million pounds in his will, you'd be pretty excited when that cheque arrived, wouldn't you? The inheritance you have in the Lord far exceeds money or riches.

—to the end that we who were the first to hope in Christ should be to the praise of His glory.

We are the praise of his glory. You can choose to be a powerful and impressive praise to his glory. You can be self-controlled and long-suffering to the praise of his glory. You can lose pounds and inches to the praise of his glory. You can remain faithful to your new way of eating no matter how long it seems to take to lose weight to the *praise of his glory*.

In Him, you also, after listening to the message of truth, the gospel of your salvation—having also believed, you were sealed in Him with the Holy Spirit of promise.

You're not just attached to Jesus with a paper clip. You're not just loosely attached to the promise of heaven. You're *sealed* in Jesus. You're sealed with the Holy Spirit of promise. There's no greater sealer than the Holy Spirit. He is eternal, all-powerful, all-knowing, wise and wonderful.

Who is given as a pledge of our inheritance, with a view to the redemption of God's own possession, to the praise of His glory.

You are God's own possession. You're sealed in him and you are his possession.

And all this time you thought you were worthless?

Reread the above verses. Write your own paraphrases

and memorize them. This is your position in Christ. You are above your circumstances. You are no longer a victim of circumstances. You're blessed with every spiritual blessing in heavenly places. Ephesians 2:6 says that you are raised up with him, seated with him in heavenly places. You're above it all!

Start acting on what you are in him.

PRAYER

In the name of Jesus, I renounce my old carnal nature. The godless passions and desires in my life are no longer going to have a hold over me. I know that they are crucified! Crucified with Christ because I am his! My mind is his, my will is his, my thoughts are his, my desires are his, my passions are his, my heart is his, my needs are his, my wants are his.

I am blessed with every spiritual blessing in heavenly places in Christ!

I am *chosen* in him before the foundation of the world!

I am predestined as an *adopted* person of his!

I am lavished with his *grace*!

I have *redemption* through his blood and *forgiveness*!

I have *wisdom* and *insight* in the name of Jesus!

He has made the mystery of *his will* known to his children!

I have obtained an *inheritance* in Christ!

I am *sealed* in him with the Holy Spirit of promise!

I am God's own possession!

In the mighty name of Jesus, Amen.

Seventeen

Why Do You Overeat?

For years Shirley blamed her overeating on her husband. If he weren't such an impossible person with so many problems, she said, she wouldn't be so nervous and frustrated and wouldn't eat so much.

Jim, a student, blamed his overeating on the pressures of college. He said he could hardly wait until he left so that he could get his eating under control. (Three weeks after leaving he put on another 10lb. He blamed it on boredom.)

Connie gained 15lb after her divorce. Tom gained 20lb when he was sent to another department at his place of work. Lorraine gained 5st with her pregnancy. Marcia gained 2st after her husband died. Every year during the holidays Denise gains between 5–10lb, and blames it on her children who, although thin, love to eat.

Why do *you* overeat?

Have you ever thought your problem was unique and separate from the rest of the world? If your slim friends had the life of troubles that you had, they'd gain weight, too, you think.

Have you ever thought nobody suffers like you do? This way of thinking says everybody has a happier and better life than *you* and eating is all you've got. The notion that others are happier, better off and leading lives of comparative ease is not true at all. There is also a mistaken belief that it's not as hard for others to lose weight as it is for you. Everyone who has ever gone on a weight-loss course has had to struggle with temptation, deny themselves and go without.

That's what it says in the word anyway. In 1 Corinthians 10:13 it says:

> No temptation has overtaken you but such as is common to man.

This verse is telling us that we are in a human realm of existence and the problems that beset us are all within this human realm. There's no superhuman task for us to undertake when we are within the confines of this realm. That's why the Lord tells us in Matthew 17:20 that if we have faith the size of a mustard seed, nothing is impossible to us.

> ...and God is faithful, who will not allow you to be tempted beyond what you are able, but with the temptation will provide the way of escape also, that you may be able to endure it (1 Cor 10:13).

With the temptation, God always provides a way of escape so that you may endure and not fall.

The reason many of us don't grab hold of this promise is because we want to be excused from our Christian responsibility to think and act like Christians.

What makes us do it?

Has anyone or anything made you angry lately? Anyone or anything made you upset, worried, furious, miserable, frustrated, depressed or anxious?

Have you ever noticed the way children behave when

they've been caught doing something they shouldn't be doing? One of the first things they might say is, 'Oh, he made me do it! Two small boys invade the biscuit tin and when Mother catches them, they both point at the other and say in unison, '*He* made me do it!'

It's the mature person who can stop blaming people and situations for his/her own sins. The responsibility for our happiness is on our own shoulders. Nobody else holds it for us.

People don't actually make you angry. You make yourself angry. Imagine driving along in your car with a friend. This friend is telling you every turn and stop to make, as if you had never been behind a wheel before. He is being a backseat driver *par excellence*.

You think to yourself, 'He is really making me angry. I'll explode in a minute.'

Explode you may, but not beause he makes you angry. You may want to throw your Grand Prix trophy at him, but please, as you do, tell the truth and say, 'I *make myself* angry when you tell me how to drive.'

Nobody else makes you anything. You make *yourself* feel, think, say, act and do what you do. Nobody else actually makes you overeat. You overeat because of you.

You *condition* yourself to eat what you eat, where you eat, how much you eat and when you eat.

What it means to be conditioned

If you have had several happy experiences when simultaneously eating and watching TV, there is an automatic trigger inside your brain that will tell you to eat when you are in front of the TV. You only need to see a TV set turned on and you'll feel like eating something. If you have paperwork to do and you've conditioned yourself to eat while working, you'll find yourself thinking of food as you work. If you have made a habit of eating when you're depressed, upset, lonely or worried, your brain will tell you to eat when you are in these states of mind. You've conditioned yourself to eat when you encounter these stressful circumstances.

Now, here's the good news. You can de-condition yourself. You can develop new habits so that your brain does not think *food* when you are in certain situations or places, or engaging in certain activities. One woman says that she doesn't overeat at all during the day when she is at work, but the minute she walks into her flat, she starts to eat and doesn't stop until she goes to bed.

Somewhere along the line she conditioned herself to think food and home are inseparable. At work she didn't think about eating, but once home, her 'eat' trigger was pulled and off she went, eating everything in sight.

Home should not mean food to us. Home is many things, and eating is only one of the things we do there. Those experiences as a child when Mother cooked up those feasts in her kitchen and all the family rallied around the table at mealtimes, may still remain in your memory. So you spend your years trying to relive these childhood experiences. Or maybe relaxation means food to you. When you arrive home after a day of pressure and hard work, you want to relax. Relaxation means food, so you not only eat, but you overeat.

You can end these lifetime patterns and develop new ones. You re-condition yourself.

Check if you do any of the following:

—eat while watching TV;
—eat while driving the car;
—eat while studying or doing paperwork;
—eat while reading;
—eat while on the job;
—eat while shopping;

—eat while preparing a meal;
—eat when cleaning up after a meal;
—eat more alone than with others;
—eat before going to bed;
—get out of bed in the middle of the night to eat;
—eat more on weekends than during the week;
—eat more at night than during the day;
—skip breakfast but gorge later on in the day.

Many books on dieting will tell you to substitute those fattening snacks you've been eating during these times for low-calorie snacks. This is acceptable, but it is not breaking the patterns that have been set up in your response system. If you really want mastery over these habits in your life, end them. For example: don't eat while watching TV—do your nails, sew, or paint something instead. Don't eat while studying or doing paperwork—a glass of water would be a good substitute. Don't eat while reading. Be good to yourself. Enjoy your book without getting fat.

The only danger in eating carrots instead of crisps as a snack is that you may eat carrots for a while, but then go back to crisps. The habit hasn't been dealt with. If you end the habit, you've got to the source of things.

You may have a string of Freudian excuses for overeating and being fat, but these don't have to keep you fat. You can change your behaviour if you really want to. It doesn't matter what your mother fed you on when you were just a toddler, or what you went without as an adolescent, or what your family eating patterns were. You can say no to those old habits and stop analysing and making excuses for them.

God says he will *provide a way of escape* for you. If you are an impulsive or compulsive eater, God will provide a way of escape. That's what it says in 1 Corinthians 10:13. He provides a way of escape for you—will you take it?

Practical help for those tough times of temptation

1. Tell your friends you're on a special eating course when they invite you for dinner. Tell them exactly what you *may* eat and what you may not. Don't use this opportunity to binge. Your friends will be happy to co-operate when they see it is important to you.

2. When you eat in a restaurant, do not examine the menu. Plan what you'll order before you get there. Think of the many healthy foods you can plan your meal from. A large salad with strips of turkey and cheese; cottage cheese; lean meat; chicken without the skin; broiled fish with no butter; a baked potato with no butter; fresh fruit. Don't use eating out as an excuse to binge.

3. Other people may not have yielded their eating habits to the Lord yet. Don't worry about them. You be the obedient one and praise the Lord that you are. If others want to eat fattening and unhealthy foods, you don't have to join them. You eat your salad and broiled fish and thank Jesus you've taken the escape he has provided for you!

4. Count your calories. Count them *before* you eat them. Be in control of things.

5. Don't buy fattening junk foods. If your family insists on these foods, let them buy them. One woman told her husband, 'Those snacks and junk foods will have to come out of the entertainment money because my grocery money must go on *food*.'

6. Cut up carrots, celery and cauliflower immediately and keep in a plastic container in the refrigerator to have some ready healthy 'fast food' on hand.

7. At church dinners, weddings and other food-orientated activities, pack your own nutritious and scrumptious eats in plastic containers and bags. Slip into the kitchen and put your food on a plate like the

others have—things like fresh fruit, cold sliced turkey, grated cheese, crisp vegetable salad.

8. You don't have to substitute chemical sweeteners for sugar, and drink artificially sweetened fizzy drinks. Drink fresh fruit juices without sugar. Praise the Lord for your health and beauty.

You are a unique and special person—a very important person. You deserve to have good things. Those good things do *not* include fattening and harmful foods.

You are his workmanship, created in Christ Jesus for good works (Eph 2:10). You are unique as a person created with his very own hands. He loves your soul, your spirit *and your body*. He knows your body. He formed you. It's important to him that it functions well.

For thou didst form my inward parts;
Thou didst weave me in my mother's womb.
I will give thanks to Thee, for I am fearfully and
    wonderfully made;
Wonderful are Thy works,
And my soul knows it very well.
My frame was not hidden from Thee,
When I was made in secret,
And skilfully wrought in the depths of the earth
(Ps 139:13–15).

You have begun your weight-loss course and you're going to lose every ounce you intend to lose. Remember that you're going to stick with it no matter how long it takes. There may be a million temptations, but he is continually providing a way of escape for you. The word of God will take first place over the thing you're tempted to eat. You'll speak the word to yourself and love it far more than that thing you almost ate.

The Lord will accomplish what concerns me (Ps 138:8).

This is your promise and your strength.

You are unique and special, but your problems are human. They are the same problems and struggles we all face. You are *never* alone when you are losing weight.

You are never alone when you are exercising self-control. Somebody else is saying no to dessert too. Someone else has found that way the Lord provides the overeater for escape—as you are discovering.

PRAYER

Dearest Lord, thank you that you did give me a way of escape from overeating. Thank you, Lord, that those things which trigger off an overeating response in me can be *ended*.

Give me the power and strength to change my overeating habits in the name of Jesus! I choose to change my overeating habits now. I receive the Lord's means of escape in the name of Jesus!

I am free from fat! I am free to be the real me as God ordained me to be free to be slim! In Jesus' name, Amen.

Eighteen

Who Says You Have to Overeat?

Elizabeth has raised a family of four boys. She, her husband and the boys are all overweight. One of her sons couldn't get into the army because of his obesity and another one was turned down for a job he wanted. (More and more companies are discovering obesity to be a health hazard and won't take on fat people.) Elizabeth broke into tears as she told how she had been deceived for years, thinking she was a good wife and mother by serving her family rich and fattening foods. She baked fresh breads and pastries nearly every week. She spent long hours in the kitchen cooking heavy, fattening meals. Actually she cooked these foods because *she* liked them. Through the years she taught her family how to like them and reinforced these likes by continuing to cook the same way, establishing a lifestyle of wrong eating for six people.

Not only was she creating a health hazard, but also a fast-growing social concern.

Drs Bruch Hannon and Timothy Lohman, two scientists from the University of Illinois at Urbana, say that we should be alerted to the energy output it takes to supply more food than overweight people need. Their figures, from a variety of federal agencies and other studies, show that if all overweight adults simultaneously went on diets to reach their optimum weights, the energy saved during the three to four-month diet period would be equivalent to 1.3 billion gallons of petrol.

Being overweight is a social problem and not only a personal concern, according to the scientists.

If all Americans, for instance, weighed the optimum weight and no more, the annual energy savings would equal three-quarters of a billion gallons of petrol, enough to run more than 900,000 cars each year or to supply the electrical needs of four metropolitan centres. These calculations are based on the amount of fossil fuel energy required to supply the extra food calories to maintain excess body fat on overweight people.

According to these studies, Elizabeth was stuffing her family's bellies and adding to the energy crisis without ever realizing what she was doing.

One of the first fears she expressed in her OV group concerned dieting and how it would affect her state of mind. She was afraid she'd be nervous, tense or easily irritated if she didn't eat the foods she was accustomed to.

That's another misconception. Being stuffed does not make you healthier or happier.

Nutrition and mental health

What you eat plays an important role in your emotional state of being. You may be fat and consuming huge amounts of food, but if you are not getting the vitamins and minerals your body requires according to your lifestyle, metabolism and body needs, you will suffer for it.

A common contributor to unnecessary weight gain is lack of understanding. If you are not conscious of food values, calorie content and nutritional benefits, you will not only remain fat, but you may be doing serious harm to your body and mind. The measure of your success is not only in losing weight, but in *keeping it off and having a healthy mind and body*.

If you are subject to periods of depression, mental confusion and other emotional problems for which you find no psychological cause, you may want to examine your diet. Evaluate what you are eating and see if you are eating a 'high-protein, moderate-carbohydrate' diet necessary for optimum mental stability. Are you getting enough vitamin B (tension reducing), potassium (easily excreted during stress periods), magnesium (vital for control of muscle tension and irritability)?

Processed cereals, white flour, and white sugar do not offer the complete range of B vitamins necessary to promote adequate food metabolism. Coffee and other caffeine beverages stimulate the insulin production and cover up fatigue. Avoid them because they hide the symptoms of low blood sugar and detract its cure.

Exercise—what's that?

It's nothing new that overweight people don't particularly love to exercise. One obese man sat in his chair watching the rain leak through the ceiling for hours before he got up to do something about it. 'Just didn't feel like moving,' he explained. He said he could sit for hours in one place, hardly moving, while his slim wife would get cramp sitting still for so long.

It isn't hard to understand why an overweight person doesn't like to exercise. It's laborious moving around a lot of extra weight. For some people it hurts! A fat person gets tired before a slim person does. He has less stamina and resistance to fatigue.

A fat person burns up more calories doing the same

amount of exercise as a slim person, because it takes more energy for him to move his extra weight. That's why grossly overweight people lose weight faster than those less overweight.

Your body has 666 skeletal muscles. Each muscle needs to be worked. You don't have to go out jogging or playing squash every day, but touching your toes once in a while wouldn't hurt. A few windmills with your arms swinging back and forth wouldn't be too demanding a couple of times a day. And a few stretches from the waist might be fun once in a while.

You don't have to overdo it.

A little at a time and easy does it are your rules of thumb. Overweight people are more discouraged than inspired by the demands of physical exercise. Ask the Lord how much you should be exercising and what kind of exercises you should be doing.

You may want to take a daily half-hour walk. Or cycle for half an hour. Perhaps joining a keep-fit class would be just the thing for you. The Holy Spirit is your guide and he won't fail you.

One thing you can count on: God doesn't want you to be worn out and racked with pain and misery through overdoing it. He loves your body and wants you to learn how to take good care of it.

Lack of exercise and weight gain can result in a sense of low self-esteem and depression. When your self-esteem is low and you feel depressed, you reach for the high-calorie undesirable foods. It's a vicious circle.

Doctors agree that proper nutrition, adequate rest and physical exercise all are needed for optimum health. Obesity is just one of the diseases caused by insufficient physical activity.

A common misbelief is that exercise or physical activity will increase the appetite. The truth is that we, on the whole, are already overeating for our energy needs. Research studies have proved that food intake actually declines as people move from low to moderate activity occupations. Strenuous exercise before a meal frequently acts to decrease appetite. Also, if exercise in a regular form is enjoyable, it will replace the inappropriate eating brought on by boredom and tension.

Most people don't relish the idea of exercising for weight loss because it takes so much to lose so little. It certainly isn't inspiring to know that you'd have to run up and down the stairs of the Empire State Building for four hours to lose 1lb of body fat.

The rule of thumb again is *slow and easy*. Don't get discouraged. A little at a time is fine! Instead of a four-hour running marathon, try something easier like walking to the shops instead of driving (that is, if you don't live eight miles from the nearest shop), or running on the spot for 30 seconds a couple of times a day. Easy!

A person could lose 9lb a year just by climbing the stairs to his/her fourth-floor office and back down four times a day.

If you are inactive, you must rigidly control your calorie intake or you will gain weight quickly. If you exercise moderately and regularly, you will not only feel better, but you'll be using up more calories.

Be good to yourself! The next time a friend suggests going out for a drink, persuade them to go for a walk with you instead.

Rather than centering your nights out around restaurants and eating, do something active like ten pin bowling, swimming, walking, jogging or playing squash, tennis or badminton. If you don't know how to do any of these things, learn. You are in charge of your circumstances. You create your own circumstances. If you've never played squash and you go for your first lesson feeling terribly self-conscious and unhappy about all the exercise involved, just tell yourself it may be difficult now, but it won't be when you're slimmer. You're getting ready for that day now by learning how to do enjoyable physical activities. You'll stay slim when you have a variety of activities to do with your new slim body.

If you live in a city and are discovering that exercise costs money, you can find cheaper ways of getting physical exercise. Walking and jogging are free. If you decide to jog, perhaps you could go with someone else, and that way you won't feel so self-conscious. You don't have to be a fine athlete to jog.

Walking is just as beneficial as jogging. It just takes longer to get where you're going. Walking is something you can do for free and it's great fun. Swing your arms, walk briskly, breathe deeply. Ah, yes, you'll wonder why you didn't do it sooner.

While waiting for your spin-dryer to finish, run on the spot for half a minute or so.

When driving the car or sitting at your desk, hold your stomach in for a count of twenty. Release and do it again. Do that a few times a day

Another good exercise is to avoid using elevators if you can walk. Stand on tiptoes and then lower your heels, up and down, up and down, five or ten times a few times a day.

You don't have to be an Olympic champion to be slim and in shape. You don't have to be 'the athletic type' to enjoy a couple of physical activities that will do you good. (How many times have you heard an overweight person shrug off exercise by saying, 'I'm just not the athletic type'?)

One of the main excuses for avoiding physical exercise is that we think it means lifting weights at the gym, or some other laborious and enervating activity.

Take it easy and enjoy your exercise. Be like the 40-year-old woman who started doing deep breathing exercises at the same time she started her weight-loss programme. As the weight fell off, she added a few more exercises. By the time she reached her goal weight (a loss of 2st), she was in better shape than when she was a teenager actively taking part in sports.

If you start slowly and if you do exercises that you enjoy, you can add more as your weight drops. Pray about the amount of exercise you get. Are you exercising your precious body enough?

PRAYER

Dear Lord, I know my body needs exercise. Show me how much exercise to do and what kind to do. I want to be a good steward of this body. I want to take care of it the best way I can. I want it to feel good, to be strong and to have plenty of energy.

I choose to exercise to the glory of God. I choose to take care of this body for the glory of God!

Now, dear Lord, give me the grace to bring you glory and honour through this body you have given me.

My life belongs to you, Lord, and I choose this day to exercise my body for you.

In Jesus' name, Amen.

Nineteen

Reaching Your Goal
and the Maintenance Course

It was for freedom that Christ set us free; therefore keep
standing firm and do not be subject again to a yoke of
slavery (Gal 5:1).

Five women stand at the front of the room, smiling.
Among them they have lost nearly 15st.

Sally says, 'I can't tell you how happy I am to at last be
able to get into the back seat of a two-door car. That's
something I couldn't do before. I was too fat.'

Karen says, 'At last I can wear something with a
waistline. And I can wear trousers. I was always too fat
to wear them before so I wore tent dresses.'

'I used to have to buy men's clothes,' says Terry.
'Men's clothes are bigger and made me feel smaller. I
could get a medium in men's clothes, but in women's
clothing I was an extra large.'

Barbara added: 'I wore a swimming costume for the
first time in ten years this week. If I ever went to the
beach before I wore shorts and a tee-shirt because I felt
too fat to wear a swimming costume. Thank God those
days are over!' Gloria tells of her delight when she was
able to take off her coat. 'I wore a coat *all* the time. In
church I never took if off. I wore a coat even if the

weather wasn't cold. Thank God, I can take it off now.'

They share how they held large bags in front of them to hide their fat, how they couldn't sit on a folding chair or cross their legs, they were unable to bend over or wear clothing with zips.

The greatest victory

What could be better than being slim? This is something many overweight people ask. What could be better than being able to sit cross-legged on the floor and then get up again without rolling over and flapping about like a porpoise? What could be better than throwing out their size 24 dresses? What could be better than buying a pair of jeans and looking like a teenager when you're in your thirties?

Here's what five women said.

Kay: 'I'm so happy to be slim but, truthfully, my greatest victory was not just in losing weight. My real victory was the one over self and my own selfish desires. I've been a selfish and demanding person all my life. I demanded from people, from God and from life. Everybody else was supposed to make me happy. Oh, the change in me has been enormous. My husband says he can hardly believe I'm the same person. He says it's like having a new wife. See, when I didn't get my own way, I'd get angry. I was angry *all* the time. And when I was angry, I ate. All the wrong foods, naturally. Losing 4st is wonderful, and through losing all that weight I've become a new person.'

Ann: 'I used to be aggressive and loud. I used to think I was extrovert, but really I was being pushy. I always felt driven to do something, be something, gain recognition, get people's attention and love. Now people are telling me they can't get over the change in me. I honestly feel a real sense of self-respect and inner contentment which I've never had before in my whole life. I know it's because of what God has done in me while losing weight.'

Jean: 'I know what you mean. I had so many problems that manifested themselves through overeating. God showed me that my overweight was not a problem that stood alone. It was due largely to my rebellion against accepting his will in my life. I wanted my way, he wanted his. Guess who loses in a tug-of-war like that! I lose if I don't obey, that's for sure. I win if I obey. I decided to obey. It wasn't easy at times. Often I thought I was being tortured needlessly and I wanted to eat something I wasn't supposed to. But I stuck to the course and now I've reached my goal. I feel better now than I have in my whole life!'

Gloria: 'Every day for a year I counted each and every calorie that went into my mouth. I didn't miss a single bite and I wrote it all down. I followed the course perfectly. I lost 6st. Now, a year may seem like a long time to count calories, but staying at my goal weight is not hard for me now because I spent a whole year developing new habits and attitudes about food. The Lord has shown me how possessive and unruly I was. My life was filled with lack of discipline and rebellion. I didn't even know it! I wanted, wanted, wanted. I was angry, hostile, spoiled and grumpy. I cry every time I think of how God has got rid of all that rubbish in my life. He did more than clean out my stomach. He cleaned out my heart and soul as well.'

It was for freedom that Christ set us free; therefore keep standing firm and do not be subject again to a yoke of slavery (Gal 5:1)

Ethel Waters, in her autobiography *To Me It's Wonderful* (Harper & Row 1972) talks about her battle with fat. She was more than 14st overweight and had lost her ability to do even ordinary things like walk or sit in a chair and get up again. Being obese had also made her bitter. She hated being fat, hated herself for being fat and hated others for reminding her she was fat.

It's no fun to be so fat that everyday activities become enormous obstacles to overcome. It's hard on the self-esteem when the seat belts in cars and aeroplanes won't go round you. Ethel Waters was humiliated and horrified when a plane she was on actually had to delay take-off until an extension belt was found long enough to go round her. When she sang in concerts she had to wear the microphone around her neck because she couldn't get close enough to a standing microphone. Her stomach was too big. She said, 'Don't laugh at a fatty. They're *handicapped*.'

'If you're fat,' she said, 'get it off, or it can kill you. I know.' She lost 14st by faithfully following her doctor's orders and praying to her heavenly Father for help. As she lost weight, she lost the bitterness and anger too. Her love for God and people grew and she became a much-loved Christian performer.

Overeating for whatever reason you can think of is *bondage*. It's like being in a prison or being wrapped in heavy chains from head to toe. You're trapped like an animal in a cage, unable to move freely. Binging and gluttony are your slave drivers. They crack the whip and you jump like a beaten and wretched slave. Whatever emotion you blame your overeating on, you are a slave to it. You may say, 'Oh dear, I'm feeling depressed. I want to eat something.'

Or, 'How dare he speak to me that way. He doesn't love me. Nobody loves me. I'm all alone in this life, loveless and lonely. I think I'll eat.'

Thoughts like these shove you right into the prison cell and shut the doors behind you. You're caught. In goes the food and out goes your stomach. Soon your stomach sticks our further than your chest and soon you can't sit with your legs together any more. Soon you find you can't be comfortable leaning back in a straight chair; you have to straddle it. You're uncomfortable in a school desk and you can't wear seat belts. You're hooked and trapped. You are indeed 'handicapped'.

Now that you've begun your eating programme, you've arrived home at last. Your body has finally emerged from that hulk you once were. The real you has popped out of these prison walls. Thank God, you're free! It was for the sake of freedom that your Saviour set you free. Praise God, keep standing firm! Don't go back to that ugly prison again!

You have victoriously feasted on Jesus and his word and reached your goal weight. The real you is now reading these words. Those hands of yours are no longer swollen and bulging around your rings, your breathing is easier and you're not gasping for breath. Your clothes fit. You feel great. Praise God, you're the real you! You are free to be slim!

Many have said, 'That fat person just wasn't me. I knew somewhere in all those extra pounds there was a real me!'

Purpose of the maintenance course

You go on the maintenance course when you reach the *spiritual goals* that God has set for you. This is the point where you are completely honest with the Lord in your life. You no longer hide calories from the Lord, you don't miss your daily 'power time', you fight those things that trigger gluttonous eating, you stop complaining about not being able to eat certain foods, you remain faithful to your calling and God's will for your body.

If you are still having temper tantrums and going on weekend binges, you're not ready for the maintenance course quite yet.

You want to maintain the good work God has done in you for the rest of your life. You don't want to prolong the fleshly indulgences and poor habits.

The reason for going on the maintenance course is so that God can continue to move in our lives, as he desires. God has a lot he wants done in our lives and he wants to get on with it! The longer you sit in fleshly indulgences, self-pity, anger, overeating, gluttony, binging and eating wrong foods, the longer it takes him to get on with the other wonderful things he has for you in your life! *Don't miss out!*

Maintaining your goal weight is God's method of keeping control of your actions and desires. You must never take this away from him.

When you begin your maintenance course there are two things that will be different at first.

You will not be counting calories in the same way any longer.

Keeping the calorie log has become second nature to most of us. Successful losers are so used to counting calories, it's hard to stop.

But you don't stop entirely. Once you reach your ideal weight and you are at the spiritual level of obedience that God wants you, you count calories two days a week—on Mondays and Fridays. On the other days, you write in your log *maintenance*. Some people notice they actually eat *less* when they ease off the calorie logging. It's because they're completely at the mercy of God and depending on him to guide and direct them.

If you can't make it without counting calories, by all

means continue. The idea is to *slowly* wean off the calorie log sheets. Don't do it all at once! If recording Monday and Friday is uncomfortable, start by eliminating just one day a week. Write *maintenance* under that day. You have self-control now. A person with self-control is ready to go on a weight maintenance course.

'But how do I know what to eat?' you may ask. You *do* know what to eat. You have been on the course long enough and listened to the voice of the Lord long enough and been in the word long enough to know very well what to eat and what not to eat. Stand firm and do not be subject again to a yoke of slavery. You are now accustomed to saying no to your own fleshly indulgence and saying yes to the Holy Spirit when he guides you in godly eating.

Ask the Lord if, what and how much you may eat. When you ask him how many caloires you ought to eat, he may very well answer, 'You know what your body needs. I have already taught you that.'

The reason you are on the maintenance course now is that you *do* understand yourself and your body and you are in *control*. Imagine spending several weeks teaching a child how to ride a bicycle. He falls a few times, makes some mistakes, but finally, he does very well. He gains co-ordination and stays on the bicycle. You can see that he has learned how to ride well. Then you tell him, 'Okay, you're ready now to go on a trip.'

He answers, 'But how do I ride the bike?'

You answer, 'I have taught you how to ride. You know how to ride. All you have to do is *do it* now.'

'But how do I do it? What do I need to know in order to ride the bicycle?'

'I have already told you everything you need to know. You have already shown me that you know how to ride the bike. You are prepared. Go ahead.'

Your calorie limit is now removed. By now you *know*

how many calories it takes to maintain your weight.

The reason God wants you to act on what you know is that he wants to teach you something new! He doesn't want you in the same old rut for ever. You have learned much about yourself and your body. Now go on! He has more for you!

Every day when you get out of bed, ask the Lord what you should eat that day. Give him your day and every morsel of food you'll be putting into your mouth.

You're on maintenance and all the more reason to *stand firm*. Fried food should be no less disgusting to you now than it was while you were losing weight. Neva Coyle didn't taste ice cream for two years. 'This is a life-long thing,' she explains. 'Things like sweets and ice cream are no friends of mine. They're not treats, either, I'll tell you that. They are *enemies*. I don't consider cakes and biscuits refreshments either. Not when I was once 17½ st. These foods are threats to my health and well-being. I choose to stand firm and not be subject again to the yoke of slavery these kinds of 'refreshments' and 'treats' once had on me. My treats are now healthy, life-giving foods, the kind my body loves, like fresh fruit, yogurt, raw vegetables and fruit juices.'

You will have a closer awareness of yourself through your diary.

Keep a very close log of your feelings, moods and behaviour at this time. Make your diary entries longer and spend more time reading the Scriptures. The reason for this is that you need to have complete control over yourself, your desires, thoughts, wants, dreams, emotions and actions. Leave nothing to chance. It was not by 'chance' you lost weight. It took concentrated effort on your part and a good deal of hard work. Don't relax your efforts now! If anything, pull *in* on the reins; don't loosen them.

In order to make your maintenance course a living reality and the joy it ought to be, go back again to making out a Desire-Action Worksheet. Write your desires and the actions you are taking to fulfil these desires. Your desire is now to maintain your goal weight. What are you doing about it?

Make this apply to other areas of your life.

Here is what one woman on the Maintenance Course wrote:

DESIRE	ACTION
Stop yelling at the kids.	Begin each day praying for each of them. Choose a special scripture verse for them and repeat these throughout the day in order to be thinking God's thoughts about my children instead of my own, which may be hurtful and selfish.
	Go to bed early so I am rested.
	Be certain their duties are clearly understood and make them aware of the punishment if they do not complete these when expected. This will eliminate my shouting at them and getting myself upset.
	Pay careful attention to our diet so we are getting plenty of the B vitamins (necessary for healthy nerves). Add more calcium, too.
	Meditate on what Jesus would do if he were in my shoes. What is his thinking on this? How does he feel about my children and about our situation? He wouldn't yell. What would he do?

This is also a good time for you to do your *God's Will for Me* chart again. You don't want to discard these practices from your life. You should continue with these charts in order to keep in close contact with *yourself*. Remember, *you* are in control of your life. These are some tools to help you stay in control. You stay in control by keeping close contact with yourself, your feelings and your actions. Your diary is of vital importance at this point.

Reach out with your new self-control in other areas of your life. You have self-control in your eating and you'll have it in other areas too.

Temptation

You won't be tempted to overeat as you once were, but you may encounter the temptation to relax your dependence on Jesus. That is why you'll have to do something to increase your dependence upon him. You may be tempted to say things like:

'Oh, one little piece of cake won't hurt me. After all, I'm at my goal weight now.'

Don't forget that it was that shelf loaded with cakes in the baker's window, the ice cream parlour, those desserts, gravies, rich and fattening foods that once tempted you to the point of your body becoming ugly! Do you want to become a prisoner of these foods again? It was for freedom that Christ set you free; therefore keep standing firm and do not be subject again to a yoke of slavery.

Make a list of the 'yokes of slavery' that once held you bound. Include the reasons why you overate too. Then write how Jesus has healed the hurts that motivated you to eat.

The truth is:

One little piece of that fattening and unhealthy food may hurt you deeply. It could start you on the habits that made you fat in the first place. You now have all the more reason to pull in the reins.

You're free to be slim for ever, not just for a little while. Now you know how to say no to yourself. Make no provision for the flesh.

The only food you deserve is the food that blesses your body and soul. The food you deserve is good, wholesome, healthy food that will make your body run the best it possibly can. You deserve the best! You are a very special child of God and your body deserves more than junk. You worked hard at losing weight. You deserve the best!

PRAYER

Father, in the name of Jesus, I am free because Jesus has set me free. I am standing firm. I will not be subject again to a yoke of slavery.

I am no longer a slave of anger, revenge, frustration, loneliness, nervousness, worry, or boredom.

I no longer eat to reward myself.

I no longer eat for comfort.

I no longer eat as a treat.

I am no longer a slave to other people's eating habits. I no longer eat unhealthy and fattening foods to please others or to avoid hurting their feelings.

I eat according to the word of God—to glorify God in my body.

I make these statements in the name of Jesus Christ, my Lord and Saviour, who redeemed me from sin and death by his own death on the cross. His blood was shed for me so that I can be free to love him and serve him with my whole body, soul and spirit.

I thank you, Father, in the name of Jesus, that I am free from overeating, free from gluttony, free from binging, free from fat *for ever*! Free to be slim.

Thank you for my maintenance course which I begin in the name of Jesus and for your glory.

In Jesus' name, Amen.

Twenty

Keeping What's Yours

Mr and Mrs Meanwell are standing at the threshold of their new home, which they have spent the last several months building. It's a life-long dream come true. They've always wanted a new house. The decorating and finishing touches are complete and they are ready to move in. They are very happy indeed.

As they stand admiring the beautiful finished result they see a storm heading their way.

They get inside the house just before the skies open and wind and rain assail the neighbourhood. What do Mr and Mrs Meanwell do next? As the storm rages outside, instead of closing all the windows and doors, they suddenly open them. They throw open the front door, back door, french windows and garage doors.

Then they watch as the rain ruins the wallpaper, carpeting and floors, and they cry, 'Oh, poor us. Everything happens to us!' Then they drag their furniture outside and set it in the mud, crying, 'Isn't this awful! Even our furniture is getting ruined in this storm.'

Far-fetched? Not really. Look at yourself for a moment. You now have a new body. It's a beautiful new home and you've worked hard for it. When storms of temptation come your way, what are you going to do? Are you going to open the doors and windows of your heart and mind for the storms to ruin? Are you going to let temptations damage any part of your beautiful new self?

If Mr and Mrs Meanwell really love their new home, they'll protect it. They'll make sure it is built well so it is able to withstand storms. They'll take care of it and be certain it is in good shape at all times. It's important because they have a big investment in it.

Your investment is even bigger. You've invested your life. If your home of bricks and mortar were to be destroyed, your body would not necessarily die because of it. You could go on living, although you'd have to find another home. But this isn't true with your body. If your body is destroyed, where else can you move? It's shocking how many people take better care of their homes than their precious bodies.

God also has an investment in you.

> When a strong man fully armed guards his own homestead, his possessions are undisturbed, but when someone stronger than he attacks him and overpowers him, he takes away from him all his armor on which he had relied, and distributes his plunder (Lk 11:21-22).

You will maintain your goal weight for ever when you keep a continual guard over your mouth and your appetite. You can't assume for a minute that because you are slim you can relax and lay your armour down. You're in this battle for good you know. By now you're an experienced soldier, the kind who leads others to the victory you've achieved.

You may want to say, but when does it all end? When can I stop being the perpetual soldier in the battlefield of life? It's tiresome to be on guard around food for ever.

It's never tiring to be in the army of God. You never get exhausted or weary when you're in the battle of the Lord with him at the front lines right beside you. He's the winner at all times. In him we live and move and have our being. So don't think for a moment that having your guard up against temptation will be a tiresome thing. It's not. It's invigorating! It energizes you. One lady who had reached her goal said, 'My husband can't get over how much energy I've got. When I was fat, I didn't have any energy; I was apathetic all the time.'

Galatians 6:9 says, 'And let us not lose heart in doing good, for in due time we shall reap if we do not grow weary.' Read that verse and then tell yourself not to lose heart in doing good. You've done well up to now. Don't be weary now, of all times. You've made it! Your body is submitted to God! You've obeyed, you've denied yourself, you've refused fleshly indulgence. Now you have a beautiful new body to glorify the Lord in. Praise God for the wisdom to stand and stay on guard!

Remember, that unruly old self of yours would love to put your wisdom to sleep, just when you need it most. There's a plate of biscuits in front of you and you haven't eaten lunch yet. What harm could one little biscuit do? (Bye-bye wisdom!) What harm could two little biscuits do? (Hello Chump!) Three? Six? After ten you lose count. Don't give me that look. It *could* happen to you. Your guard is your friend. Love yourself. Love your wisdom and your integrity. You're a beautiful new you now. You're no longer a chump for a plateful of biscuits. Your taste is fixed on higher things. Let the fat people eat the biscuits. You feast on the word of God and *pray* for the fat people.

'Put on the full armour of God' it says in Ephesians 6. Now why does a person have to go around with the full armour of God on anyway? Isn't that tiring? I mean, a person could think of better things to do than haul around a heap of armour all day and night, couldn't he?

No, a person could not. Don't just put on the armour of God; put on the *full* armour of God—all of it. Satan's schemes are to get you fat again, steal your victory, make you miserable. He hates God and he hates you. He wants to wreck anything that glorifies God. He'd like to break every bone in your body—destroy you completely. He'd like to turn you into a piece of mud and get you to curse God. He hates it that you're not fat and ugly any more. He hates it that you *like* yourself now.

Do you see why we are talking about the *full* armour of God?

> For our struggle is not against flesh and blood, but against the rulers, against the powers, against the world forces of this darkness, against the spiritual forces of wickedness in the heavenly places (Eph 6:12).

But *how* do you put on the full armour of God? It's relatively simple. You stay completely honest with the Lord. You remain in complete and continual communication with him. Stand firm, therefore, having girded your loins with truth. Gird means to encircle or bind with a belt or band. It means to surround; hem in. That's what we are to do with the truth—bind ourselves to it and in it. He is truth.

Connect yourself to heaven on a direct line that is used continually to talk to him. Praise him, worship him. Keep reading the word. And listen when he speaks to you.

'When I begin to stumble it's because I'm not in the word,' say one person who lost 4st. Again and again the same is heard from hundreds of successful weight losers.

'When I'm not in the word, I'm liable to gain weight.

I'm liable to overeat.'

'It's always when I'm not faithful in reading the word that I eat what I shouldn't. When I pray every day and ask the Lord to show me what to eat, when I meditate on the Scriptures and speak the living word to myself, I don't blow it. I stand strong and girded.'

So will you!

You need your daily 'power time' like you need air to breathe and water to drink. You need it like you need rest and food. You need it like you need life to live.

...*having put on the breastplate of righteousness*. The breastplate is your spiritual shield over your heart. Your heart is hypothetically the centre of your being, the well from which spring your emotions, conscience, desires, dreams and affections. Wear righteousness like integrity.

One woman who lost over 7st went to a café with her husband. He was accustomed to eating gooey sundaes with whipped cream on top. He asked her to join him in his indulgence. She thought, 'Well, why not? I can afford *one* scoop of ice cream[1] at 150 calories a scoop...' Her breastplate of righteousness was still in place, in spite of these dangerous words. She had been on her weight-loss course for over a year. She had developed

[1] Have you been telling yourself that ice cream is nutritious because it's a supposed milk product? Here are just a few of the more than 60 chemical additives that might be inside your favourite ice cream: carrageenan, furcelleran, agar-agar, alcin, calcium sulfate, gelatin, gum karaya, locust bean gum, oat gum, gum tragacanth, mono-and diglycerides, polysorbate 65 and 80, sodium carboxymethylcellulose, propylene glycol alginate, microcrystalline cellulose, dioctyl sodium sulfosuccinate, sodium citrate, disodium phosphate, tetrasodium pyrophosphate, sodium hexametaphosphate, calcium carbonate, magnesium carbonate, calcium oxide and hydroxide, magnesium oxide and hydroxide. These additives are used to simulate flavour, colour, texture and to prevent crystal formation during storage. Ice cream does not list ingredients on the package. This high-calorie dessert, loaded with sugar, just isn't what you think it is.

new patterns, even though her old hungry nature was rearing its head in this tempting situation.

She picked up the menu and began to read—something she had stopped doing long ago. She was well aware of the pitfalls of reading a menu. Menus make the worst things sound delicious. Some of them even show pictures of the foods, deadly for the overeater.

She read the descriptions of every concoction. When the waitress came to take their order, her husband ordered his gooey mess and she said, as if automatically programmed, 'I'll have tea, please.'

When you are ready spiritually to go on the maintenance part of your weight-loss course you are no longer *developing* beautiful eating habits, you're *living* them. This woman was not accustomed to eating ice cream. At one time in her life her affections were set on such things as this. Now her affections were totally possessed by Jesus. Maintaining your goal weight means to reap the benefits of the weight-loss habits you have sown.

Having shod your feet with the preparation of the gospel of peace.
You're no longer stumbling around confused or bewildered. You're walking in the Spirit now! You're wise, able to make right choices! You're good to yourself. Can you praise the Lord right now as you are reading this and thank him for your walk in the Spirit?

You are a partaker of his divine nature!

You have crucified the desires and passions of the flesh!

You are walking in the Spirit and your feet are wearing the truth of the word of God!

Your shield of faith extinguishes all the flaming missiles of the evil one.

Every day when you have your daily 'power time' and you pray to the Lord about your appetite, you are exercising faith. The Lord loves your faith. It's impossible to please him without faith (Heb 11:6). When you trust him to help you with your problem of overeating, you are exercising faith that will indeed help.

The cry of so many overeaters is, 'How can I be a good witness for Jesus when I'm so overweight? How can I tell people that Jesus will help them with their problems when my own weight problem is so obvious?'

One woman named Sharon wrote these tragic words on a response sheet:

'One night in March of this year I was at work and talking with some of the ladies. One of them was really concerned about her husband and the terrible way he treated his health. Then she started putting down everybody who smoked and drank. Well, when she left the room, the other ladies just exploded. They said, "She's got a nerve talking about how other people harm their bodies when she's so *fat*." I shrank in my chair because I was 5ft 2in and weighed 14st. These ladies knew I was a Christian and I was suddenly so ashamed of myself. I had put down people who smoked and drank too. Here I was, no better than they were. I was killing my own body by overeating.'

Then Sharon stopped feeling sorry for herself and picked up her shield of faith. She lost 2st by the end of July. The fellowship she found with other Christians who were learning how to carry their shields of faith was the help and encouragement she needed. 'I had just never considered before that God could be my strength in this area of my life,' she explains.

The ladies at work didn't know how much an impact their words had on her that day back in March. They see the change in her now though. They see that Jesus is making a difference in Sharon's life and that he is a big enough Lord to help her become slim.

Being overweight should never stop anyone from telling others about the love of Jesus! He heals us of all

our diseases, delivers us from destruction and is the
Saviour of mankind. He saves us from overeating!

*...take the helmet of salvation, and the sword of the
Spirit, which is the Word of God.*

One relatively new person to the OV course had a
hair-raising experience as she was travelling along the
motorway one day. She saw on the seat beside her an
almost-empty packet of biscuits her children had left
there. She hadn't had any breakfast and so she absent-
mindedly reached over and took one of those biscuits.
After she had eaten about six of them her appetite was
such that she could have eaten anything in sight. She
decided she had enough time to stop at a service station
and eat breakfast.

She'd have the whole lot, she decided, since she was
so hungry. She pulled off the motorway at the next
service station. She was practically breathless as she
pulled into the car park. She knew what the menu
looked like with all those photos of tempting dishes.
She could see the rows and rows of foods listed, she
could almost smell the bacon frying in the kitchen. She
jumped out of the car and walked towards the entrance.
Suddenly she heard within her the Bible verse, 'Having
begun with the Spirit, are you now ending with the
flesh?' She stopped in her tracks. Her feet, although she
didn't think so, were still shod with the gospel of peace.
The word of God was still her mighty sword.

'I don't have to do this thing,' she told herself. 'I can
get back into my car and stop this binge before it starts.'

Those biscuits had triggered off a food-lust response
in her and she could have eaten enough food for six
people. Obviously, she wouldn't have wisely ordered a
boiled egg (you don't eat wisely when you're binging).
She would have eaten like a monstrous human dustcart.
She knew it and so did the Lord.   It was the word that
stopped her—*the word of God!*

Soak in the word of God so it can hold you tightly and guard you from yourself. The sword of the Spirit will slice apart and tear into shreds every plot to make you binge and get fat again.

She rushed back to her car and arrived at her destination early. There she had her daily quiet time with Jesus, feasting on a magnificent spiritual meal. What a wonderful victory.

PRAYER

Dear Jesus, I choose to allow nothing to interfere with my relationship with you and the teaching you have brought into my life regarding eating. I completely cover myself in the armour of God so that I am able to resist temptation and stand my ground. I tighten the belt of truth around my waist. I put on the breastplate of righteousness and integrity. I shoed my feet in preparation by reading and meditating daily on your word. I lift up the shield of faith which comes by reading the Bible. I quench the flaming missiles of Satan in your wonderful name.

Dear Jesus, I choose the helmet of salvation. I take the sword of the Spirit, which is the word of God. I choose to pray at all times in the Spirit, and keep alert to those things which could destroy me.

I pray this way, dear Lord, to affirm my commitment to you and to exercise my inheritance as a child of God. In Christ I am victorious.

Amen.

Twenty-one

How to Talk About Losing Weight Without Being an Unbearable Bore

What could be worse than being excited about something, sharing it with your friends and discovering you're boring them to tears? You may wonder what's wrong with everybody. Why don't they find the same fascination in discussing my lunch as I do? Where is the drum roll when I talk about how I *never* eat my veg with butter or margarine?

Why doesn't everybody else jump for joy when I announce I'm 1¾ lb lighter than I was this very minute last Tuesday?

Not only are people who talk endlessly about their diet bores to other people, they are usually self-styled trumpeters for the stomachs of the world. You wouldn't dare eat a baked potato in front of some dieters (even though you'd wisely omitted the butter and dolloped a tablespoon of cottage cheese on top) because they would give you that insidious blank expression that says, 'Good grief, are you really going to eat *that?*' until you lost your appetite.

You're an Overeater Victorious. You've got it together. People need only look at you to see that you're free from the bondage of fattening and unhealthy food.

You don't need to glare at someone about to eat a

greasy hamburger or get on a soap box to preach against the sins of gluttony at the next opportunity.

People will not only be observing a slimmer you, they will clearly observe a happier you. This is because when a person lives in obedience to God, he becomes a happier person. There's no happier place to be than in obedience to the will of God.

You knew from the beginning that your overeating was a spiritual problem. This is humbling. You don't ever want this divine liberating knowledge to turn sour in your heart by pointing an accusing finger at other fat people. Have mercy on them and have compassion. Have compassion on yourself too.

The only way to share the love and goodness of the Lord is to do it in love. Jesus doesn't throw poisoned darts at obese people. He says, 'Come unto me, all you who are heavy laden...' He doesn't condemn and turn his back on those who eat the wrong foods. He says simply, '*I* am the bread of life!'

Eating healthy foods shouldn't become doctrine. Primary doctrine must always be Christ crucified, risen and coming again. He came to set us free, and we must take care not to tie ourselves into knots over the evils of unhealthy food in the world. 'Be *wise* as serpents, *harmless* as doves,' he tells us.

Love is something you *do*. You *do* act kindly. You *do* encourage others. You *do* give your time and energy to help someone else. You *do* act as though other people's bodies are as important as your own.

One woman had been attacking alcoholics for years until she realized 1 Corinthians 3:16–17 pertained to her as well as the alcoholics of the world. 'Do you not know that you are a temple of God, and that the Spirit of God dwells in you?' These words inspired her to lose 4½st of fat.

Losing weight and changing your eating habits for

the glory of God gives you a merciful and an understanding heart towards others. It never makes you
judgemental, accusing or haughty

> For the whole law is fulfilled in one word in the statement,
> 'You shall love your neighbour as yourself (Gal 5:14).

I AM VICTORIOUS

Today I walk in victory. I am totally victorious over
food. I do not abuse food or use it for satisfaction,
reward or emotional outlet. I do not express my anger
or frustration by overeating.

Jesus alone satisfies me. Jesus alone gives me strength
to handle anger, frustration, and to live up to my daily
responsibilities. I need no other reward than to walk in
a covenant of obedience with him. He is God, my
Father. He is my Saviour in the person of Jesus Christ.
He is my helper in the person of the Holy Spirit.

I worship God today in obedience, praise and posi-
tive attitudes. I am loved by God. I also love and respect
myself. Jesus died for me and has forgiven all my sins. I
am entitled to the best of life because Jesus died to give
it to me.

I have put off the works of the flesh and clothed
myself in the righteousness of Christ. The Holy Spirit
empowers me to be free *not* to eat the foods that make
me fat. I will be slim in the name of Jesus and for his
glory.

He is mine and I am his completely. I use the word of
God as my weapon for battle. I fight winning battles
and do not surrender to junk foods and the works of the
flesh. I choose to walk in the Spirit by the power of God
which infuses in me.

I am victorious!

Twenty-two

Food for Thought

Usually an overweight person wants to be much slimmer than he really ought to be. A woman who now weighs 29½st dreams of weighing a mere 7½st one day. The thought of it is so impossible and exhausting to her she runs to the cake tin for something to eat to 'calm her nerves'. Perhaps the Lord's ideal weight for her is 10st 5lb, which is still a long way off, but not quite so far off as 7½st.

To maintain your weight at 7½st you would eat no more than 1,680 calories a day. If your ideal weight is 10st 5lb you would eat no more than 2,320 calories a day in order to maintain that weight.

Here's how it works. Decide on your ideal weight (after consultation with the Lord). Calculate the number of pounds, and multiply that by 16.

Example: Your ideal weight is 9st 9lb (which is 135lb). Multiply by 16 and you get 2,160. That's how many calories you can consume a day to *maintain* your ideal weight.

You're not losing any weight yet though. In order to lose 1lb of stored fat, you have to omit 4,000 calories somewhere in your diet. If your 'maintaining' calorie allowance is 2,160 calories a day and you eat only 1,000 calories a day, you have cut out 8,120 calories a week. When you do that, you will have lost over 2lb! In a month's time you will drop almost 10lb.

Many dieters don't have a solid understanding of these facts. It's easy to remember them, though, if you (1) multiply your ideal weight by 16 for the calories you'll eat a day to *maintain* that weight, (2) subtract the number of calories you are now eating each day to lose weight, and (3) work out how much you'll be losing by the 4,000 calories = 1lb formula.

More 'Free To Be Slim' helps!

Soft drinks

Try replacing your soft drinks with fruit juices. Discover the beauty of plain water! You'd be amazed at how happy children can be with a glass of water when they're thirsty.

Tea and coffee

Some people think tea is healthier to drink than coffee. Actually, commercial tea contains caffeine just as coffee does. It also has tannic acid in it, harmful to your health. Another deception is that decaffeinated coffee is better for you than regular coffee. But the National Cancer Institute in America announced that the chemical, trichloroethylene or TCE, used in making decaffeinated coffee, causes cancer in the liver of mice. It served a warning of a possible cancer danger to humans.

Instant tea (not tea leaves—often found in machines) contains malto dextrin, citric acid, artificial colour and flavour, vegetable oil and BHA (a preservative). Ouch!

Hot chocolate and cocoa

Chocolate and cocoa contain caffeine from the cocoa

bean. Prepared cocoa mixes are loaded with unwanted additives.

Herb teas

Drink herb teas in moderation. There are dozens to choose from and you'll soon love them. Carry a packet of herb teabags in your bag for quick hot drinks when you are out. Just ask the waiter or your host for a cup of hot water, and you instantly have a refreshing drink. You no longer have to put coffee, tea or fizzy drinks into your precious body.

The fear of foods

You are not bound to a list of *never to be eaten foods*. You're free to eat the foods you know to be good for your body. As Christians we must not allow fear to have any part in our lives. This includes the area of food. We choose to *bless* our bodies at all times. Fear never motivates us, love does. We're not afraid of the food we eat; we're in *control* of it.

Eating healthily is easier on the budget

You *can* afford healthy food! A bag of apples is less expensive than a block of ice cream. Fresh fruit and natural foods are actually less expensive when you consider the price of many convenience foods. You'll be saving on your food bills when you eat healthy natural foods. It's a fact.

Snacks

If you've had enough for the day, don't even nibble on the carrots and celery in the refrigerator. Your body doesn't need carrots and celery if it's had its fill, so there's no reason to nibble on any food, even if it is low-calorie. That may sound cruel, but your body will thank you for it. You're in control!

Oils

Do keep oil in your diet. Use safflower oil. Use it in your salad dressings. Mix one tablespoon with lemon juice or apple cider vinegar and whatever seasonings you like. Safflower oil is a good source of lecithin, vitamin E and linoleic acid, all necessary to keep you young and energetic. The oil will help prevent water retention in your tissues and will also aid in losing weight by causing your body to change sugar to fat at a slower rate. The oil in your diet lessens your cravings for sweets and prevents hunger pangs because it causes food to remain in your stomach longer. Do not omit oil from your diet, but do not substitute animal fat, grease or other oils for safflower oil.

Eating out

Remember, don't read the menu when you go to a restaurant. *Plan ahead* what you'll order before you get there. If you're not sure the restaurant serves food you can eat, phone them first. Ask if they serve salads, vegetables without butter, seafood without batter or breadcrumbs, lean meats, fresh fruits. Most restaurants are glad to be helpful. If you're going to a dinner or some other function where the food is already prepared and you'll be expected to eat what is served, pray before going, 'Lord, let there be something there I can eat.' There will usually be something you can eat without piling on the calories. Don't even look at the dessert. Give it to the person sitting next to you or simply refuse it. Don't eat your meal staring at a dessert. You don't hate yourself any more.

Artificials and chemicals

Avoid foods with artificial sweeteners, chemicals, preservatives, artificial *any* thing. We'll get you healthy yet.

Sugar and your children.

The younger your children are, the easier it can be to eliminate sugar from their diet. William Duffy, the author of *Sugar Blues* (Warner Books 1975) says that if children are raised completely without sugar, when they are exposed to the multiple temptations of a sugared culture, they will have developed natural immunity. Given sugar, sweets or sweetened soft drinks, they reject them. Don't feed the baby sugared baby foods and sugared drinks. Low blood sugar, or eating too much sugar, produces the following symptoms in children as well as in adults: overeating, loss of memory, nightmares, bedwetting, sleepwalking, hyperactivity, nervousness, irritability, lethargy and mental fatigue. It has long been known that sugar caused hyperactivity in children. Omit sugar from the diet of your child and your child will be healthier, and probably happier, have fewer colds and infections and many even do better at school.

The human body has no nutritional need for refined table sugar. It has been linked to almost every major disease from diabetes and heart ailments to cancer. Sugar is added to tinned soups, sauces, tinned vegetables, baked beans, table salt, pickles, processed meats, rice mixtures, peanut butter, crackers—virtually *all* convenience foods.

When you read labels, be aware that these words mean harmful sugar: dextrose, sucrose, fructose, maltose, lactose and even the word carbohydrate. If you want to be sure the product you buy has no sugar, look for the words 'No sugar added'.

Raw sugar, brown sugar

Sorry, these are no better than refined white sugar. Raw sugar is simply the dirty sugar before it's further refined.

Foods to be shared

Some foods are foods to be shared. There are too many calories in them for one person alone. An avocado is such a food. It is meant to be shared because one person shouldn't eat all those 275 calories alone.

Measure foods

Don't panic. You won't have to carry the scales around and a set of measuring cups in your handbag. You need to get acquainted with what half a cup of something looks like though. If 1½oz of parmesan cheese has 170 calories, you'll need to know what it *looks* like before you can count it. One woman was shocked when she saw what half a cup of peas looked like on her plate. You must measure your food for at least three weeks. In three weeks' time you should know what certain measurements look like. Keep your scales and cups handy to check with periodically after that.

Steaming food

A delicious way to serve vegetables is to steam them. Buy a steamer to set in your pan, add approximately an inch of water to the bottom of the pan and you'll have delicious, crisp and tasty vegetables. You don't even need to add butter.

Enjoy your food

Don't take the fun out of eating. Eating is no sin. Gluttony is sin. Craving is sin. Disobedience is sin. Enjoying what God gives you blesses him. That's one of the reasons why we thank him for our daily bread. He gives it to us to bless our bodies. It's proper to enjoy what he gives us. For the overweight person, enjoyment of food has been like a god. *That* is sin. For you eating is no longer sin—it's stewardship of your body. It's the means God is using to show you obedience, love and discipline so that you will have a fulfilled and beautiful life in Christ.

Here is a simplified guideline for you to use in your food plan. Be sure to eat from every food category or group to ensure you're getting the proper vitamins, minerals and protein for each day. You are the one responsible to the Lord for what you are eating and how much each day. You adjust the portions of each food group to fit into your daily calorie allowance. You do not cut out one type of good nutritious food group to allow yourself more in another food group. You are a responsible self-controlled person. You eat in balance.

OVEREATERS VICTORIOUS RECOMMENDED DIET GUIDELINE—THE SIMPLE WAY TO EAT

Breakfast:
  High Vitamin C fruit
  Protein food—choose one
    2oz cottage or pot cheese
    1oz hard cheese
    2oz cooked or canned fish
    1 egg
    8oz cup skimmed milk
  Whole grain bread or cereal
  Beverage

Lunch:
  Protein food—choose one
    2oz fish, poultry or lean meat
    4oz cottage or pot cheese
    2oz hard cheese
    1 egg
    2 level tablespoons peanut butter
  Whole grain bread
  Vegetables–raw or cooked

Fruit—1 serving
Beverage

Dinner:
Protein food—choose one
4oz cooked fish, poultry or lean meat
Vegetables—cooked or raw
High Vitamin A
Potato
Other vegetables—you may eat freely
Fruit—1 serving
Beverage

Other daily foods:
Fat—choose 3 daily
Milk—2 cups (8oz each) skimmed

Remember: measure quantities of each serving and count every calorie.

PRAYER

Lord Jesus, help me to use these helps to the glory of God. I choose to be a faithful steward of my body. I shall faithfully measure and count the calories I put into my body. I shall become the person you have intended me to be since the beginning of time. I choose a walk of obedience, mercy, love and discipline. Thank you, Lord, for being my enabler, my strength, my motivator, my true love, my friend, my comforter, my King of kings and my Lord, Amen.

Postscript

Tomorrow

'Can you help my friend?' asked the voice on the other end of the line. 'If she doesn't lose weight, she's going to die.'

'What do you mean, she's going to die?'

The answer was strained but emphatic. 'She weighs 37½st!'

Her name is Helen and she is 28st overweight. Her doctor has told her that her heart is going to give out if she keeps gaining. Already, her breathing is laboured and difficult and her heartbeat irregular.

Her obesity has caused her to lose the use of her legs. She is confined to a wheelchair and rarely leaves her home. The only clothes she owns are a couple of enormous tent dresses large enough to drape across her body. The rolls and rolls of fat rubbing against themselves have given her running sores which do not heal. Her skin, releasing toxins and poisons, causes her home to reek with putrid, foul smells.

Where is hope? She wants to know. She has been considering a bypass operation where her intestines would be sealed off so that the food she eats will pass right through the bowels twenty minutes after she's eaten. But she's afraid of the surgery and doesn't want it—it would be dangerous anyway, bearing in mind the state of her heart and lungs.

Everything she has tried, including pills, injections, diets, even hypnosis and fasting, has not worked. She can't get out of her home to attend the many diet clubs and weight-loss groups available because moving is so laborious. It's difficult to get into a car and she is too fat to walk. Her doctor and friends know she'll die if she doesn't lose weight.

With 28st to lose, Helen needs a miracle!

She is desperate and will even give Jesus a try.

An OV leader visited Helen with her Bible and OV materials. The 37½st woman said, 'I know Jesus is my last and only hope.' She gave her heart to him and prayed with her new friend (who had lost 5st and was still losing).

Immediately prayer requests were made for Helen. Her fellow weight-losers have her name up on their refrigerator doors, bathroom mirrors, office walls, in their wallets and other places to remind them of her and to pray for her throughout the day. She is not alone in her battle against 28st too many. Others are standing with her.

Helen began to lose weight and in three weeks lost 2st. She knows it will be a long-term process. She's planning a three-year course, but she is willing to work at it. In Christ, she has found her miracle.

It is to the Helens of this world and every one of us who has ever struggled with fat that Jesus reaches his loving arms out in help and love.

PRAYER

Lord Jesus, I know you love me whatever shape I'm in, but I thank you with my whole heart that I am free to have self-control and a slim body now.

I choose to be fair and healthy as you tell me to be. I choose to be disciplined and slim in the name of Jesus. Thank you, Jesus, for setting me free to be slim. Amen.

God's Chosen Fast

by Arthur Wallis

Having proved over many years the great value and blessing of fasting, Arthur Wallis has written this book to share with us what the Bible says about this important and neglected subject. His aim is to deal not only with all the main passages in Scripture that touch on the matter, but also with the practical issues involved.

This is a balanced study which seeks to give to the subject the weight that Scripture gives it and to avoid exaggeration and over-emphasis. The book includes a biblical index, and an appendix dealing with the textual problems surrounding four references to fasting in the New Testament.

K
Kingsway Publications

God Wants You Whole
The Way to Healing, Health and Wholeness

by Selwyn Hughes

If God is always willing to heal, why do people remain ill—even when they have faith for healing?

How can we all live more healthy lives, day by day?

With openness and honesty, Selwyn Hughes faces squarely the issues of health and healing that concern every one of us. He examines the most common causes of ill health and the reasons we fail to receive God's healing grace. Here we see how our Creator has lovingly provided all we need for wholeness of living, if only we set ourselves to live in accordance with his will.

Above all, this book shows that even when healing eludes us and our condition is not remedied quickly, we can still rest secure in the knowledge that our heavenly Father is committed to our good—in spirit, mind, emotions, and body.

Also by Selwyn Hughes in Kingsway paperback:
A friend in Need; How to Live the Christian Life; The Christian Counsellor's Pocket Guide; Everyday Reflections; A New Heart; Marriage as God Intended.

Kingsway Publications